Madhu Agrawal, PhD

Global Competitiveness in the Pharmaceutical Industry
The Effect of National Regulatory, Economic, and Market Factors

Pre-publication
REVIEWS,
COMMENTARIES,
EVALUATIONS . . .

"We are now living in a global economy and there is an increasing need for valuable literature that can help us understand the various aspects of the rapidly changing world scene. In this effort, we should not ignore the important area of global pharmaceutical marketing. In this area, where there are only a limited number of good reference sources, this book is very timely and will no doubt serve as a wonderful addition. My compliments and thanks to Professor Madhu Agrawal for bringing to existence this very well-researched and well-written book that will be of immense use not only to professionals involved in pharmaceutical marketing, but also to students and scholars who are interested in learning more about the intricacies of the global pharmaceutical industry. Professor Agrawal has also done an excellent job of presenting the research findings of a great study in a manner that is easy to read and understand. Most important, this book maintains the interest of the reader."

Ashish Chandra, MMS, MBA, PhD
Assistant Professor
of Pharmacy Administration,
Xavier University of Louisiana,
New Orleans, LA

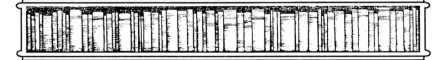

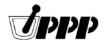

Pharmaceutical Products Press
An Imprint of the Haworth Press, Inc.

Global Competitiveness in the Pharmaceutical Industry

The Effect of National Regulatory, Economic, and Market Factors

PHARMACEUTICAL PRODUCTS PRESS
Pharmaceutical Sciences
Mickey C. Smith, PhD
Executive Editor

Global Competitiveness in the Pharmaceutical Industry
The Effect of National Regulatory, Economic, and Market Factors

Madhu Agrawal, PhD

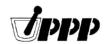

Pharmaceutical Products Press
An Imprint of the Haworth Press, Inc.
New York • London • Oxford

Published by

Pharmaceutical Products Press®, an imprint of The Haworth Press, Inc., 10 Alice Street, Binghamton, NY 13904-1580

Cover design by Jennifer M. Gaska.

Library of Congress Cataloging-in-Publication Data

Agrawal, Madhu.
    Global competitiveness in the pharmaceutical industry : the effect of national regulatory, economic, and market factors / Madhu Agrawal.
       p. cm.
    Includes bibliographical references and index.
    ISBN 0-7890-0715-0 (alk. paper)
    1. Pharmaceutical industry. 2. Drugs—Marketing. 3. Competition, International. I. Title.
HD9665.5.A353 1999
338.4'76151—DC21
                                                      99-13600
                                                           CIP

To Sanjay, Nitya, and Divya

ABOUT THE AUTHOR

Madhu Agrawal, PhD, is an Assistant Professor in the College of Pharmacy at St. John's University in Jamaica, New York. In 1997 and 1998, she received the Faculty Merit Award from the University. Dr. Agrawal is a member of the American Pharmaceutical Association and the American Association of Pharmaceutical Scientists. Dr. Agrawal's research interests include strategies in the global pharmaceutical industry, comparative studies of prescription drug advertising in different countries, consumer behavior regarding pharmaceutical products, and multicultural aspects of pharmacy practice. In addition, she has publications in journals such as *Health Marketing Quarterly, International Marketing Review, Journal of Research in Pharmaceutical Economics, Journal of Products and Brand Management, International Journal of Pharmacy Practice, Journal of Pharmacy Teaching, Journal of Transnational Management Development,* and others. Dr. Agrawal has given numerous presentations at national meetings.

CONTENTS

Preface

National competitiveness has become one of the central pre-occupations of government and industry in every nation, especially in the United States. The competitiveness of the U.S. economy in the global market became a growing concern during the 1980s due to sustained deterioration in the U.S. trade deficit. The loss of market share in products such as microelectronics, an industry thought invulnerable to foreign competition, began to raise questions regarding the overall international competitiveness of the U.S. economy.

In 1990, the U.S. Senate Committee on Finance identified three industries that were important for future U.S. competitiveness in the global economy. The committee directed the U.S. International Trade Commission to conduct investigations on these three advanced-technology manufacturing industries, one of which was the pharmaceutical industry.

The global pharmaceutical industry is a multinational industry that is highly regulated, capital intensive, and driven by large R&D expenditures. The world market for pharmaceuticals in 1996 was estimated to be U.S. $296.4 billion (*Scrip Magazine,* 1997). Supported by an ever-increasing demand for health care, world production of pharmaceuticals has grown at an exceptional pace throughout most of the postwar period. World consumption doubled between 1975 and 1990, with the world's per capita consumption of drugs increasing almost 70 percent in the same years. Very few industries can boast of such an impressive growth record.

The main objective of the research presented in this book is to examine the determinants of global competitive advantage in the ethical[1] pharmaceutical industry. Specifically, there were three main research questions:

1. Which country factors stimulate or inhibit a nation's pharmaceutical industry to be globally innovative?

2. Which country factors stimulate or inhibit diffusion of pharmaceutical innovations (NCEs)[2] into its markets?
3. Are there differences between industrialized and developing countries with respect to factors that affect innovation and global competitiveness in the pharmaceutical industry?

The above research questions were developed after a review of the literature, talking to industry experts, and from the responses of an executive survey carried out to determine the factors affecting global competitiveness in the pharmaceutical industry.

This research makes several theoretical, empirical, and methodological contributions. In addition, the results also generate important managerial and public policy implications. Theoretical contributions are made to several streams of literature on national competitiveness, pharmaceutical innovation and diffusion, economic development, and global strategic management. Significant empirical contributions the global competitiveness research on the pharmaceutical industry are made because this study uses a far larger sample of countries, a more comprehensive model, and greater sophistication in its statistical method of analysis than previous studies on this topic.

There are many managerial implications from the study results. Strategic management issues are discussed both from the perspective of industrialized country multinational corporations (MNCs) and developing country MNCs. These implications are discussed with respect to the type of core competencies that global pharmaceutical firms should develop, the various types of comparative advantages of countries that firms should exploit to develop competitive leverage, and the strategic choices that firms should make when collaborating with international firms.

Public policy implications are extremely important, because the pharmaceutical industry is heavily regulated in most countries and such regulations have far-reaching impact on its competitiveness. Public policy implications with respect to the economic environment, the regulatory environment, and the market/industry environment for pharmaceuticals are explored on the basis of the study results. Recommendations for industrialized and developing country policymakers are made with respect to their pharmaceutical industries in the global economy.

This book has five chapters. Chapter 1 presents an overview of the nature of global competition in the pharmaceutical industry and discusses its evolution in the post-World War II period. Chapter 2 reviews the literature on national competitiveness, global pharmaceutical competitiveness, and global strategic management. Studies from these streams of literature are reviewed to develop the constructs and hypotheses used in the research. Chapter 3 presents the research questions, the statistical models and statistical technique, and the constructs, measures, and data sources used in the study. Hypotheses developed to analyze the relationships are also discussed. In Chapter 4, results from the global innovation and global diffusion models are discussed, and indirect effects are examined. The results of the two-group analysis of industrialized (I) and developing (D) country groups are also discussed. Chapter 5 presents the summary of results; managerial and public policy implications of the study results; theoretical, empirical, and methodological contributions of the study; limitations of the study; and prospects for the global pharmaceutical industry in the future.

Chapter 1

The Global Pharmaceutical Industry

PRESENT STATUS AND ENVIRONMENT

The global pharmaceutical industry is a multinational industry that is highly regulated, capital intensive, and driven by large R&D expenditures. The industry is primarily privately owned and is technologically sophisticated.

The worldwide pharmaceutical market in 1996 reached U.S. $296.4 billion, up by 4 percent over 1995. (*Scrip Magazine*, 1997). The largest pharmaceutical market for 1996 was North America—it accounted for 35 percent of the world market, followed by Europe, which captured 29 percent of the market share. The ten leading pharmaceutical markets from January through September 1997 by country were: the United States, Japan, Germany, France, Italy, the United Kingdom, Spain, Canada, the Netherlands, and Belgium. Table 1.1 shows the ten leading markets in 1997, along with their estimated retail sales and percentage growth over the previous year.

Of the twenty leading companies worldwide in pharmaceutical sales for 1996/1997, nine were U.S.-based, eight were from Europe, and two were from Japan. Merck & Co. of the United States was the leading pharmaceutical company worldwide in prescription pharmaceutical sales for 1996/1997.

The leaders in this industry continue to be those countries where modern pharmaceutical production first emerged: Belgium, France, the former West Germany, Italy, Japan, the Netherlands, Sweden, Switzerland, the United Kingdom, and the United States. The pharmaceutical industry in developing countries accounts for a fifth of the world production. China is the largest producer among the developing countries, accounting for two-fifths of this group's total in 1988 (Ballance, Pogany, and Forstner, 1992).

1

TABLE 1.1. Leading Pharmaceutical Markets for 1997

Market	Jan.-Sept. 1997 Retail Sales (U.S. $ million)	Growth (%)
United States	65,990	+15
Japan	43,441	−10
Germany	14,917	0
France	14,128	+3
Italy	8,753	+7
United Kingdom	7,526	+8
Spain	4,893	+8
Canada	3,997	+9
Netherlands	1,907	+6
Belgium	1,856	+4

Source: Scrip Magazine (1998). "Steady Growth for World Pharmaceutical Sales," Scrip's Review of 1997, PJB Publications, Sussex, UK.

World consumption of pharmaceutical preparations (in constant 1980 U.S. dollars) was $70 billion in 1975, but had more than doubled to $150 billion by 1990. However, more than 70 percent of all pharmaceuticals are sold in developed market economies. The developing countries account for less than a fifth. Drug usage is growing most rapidly in Japan and North America. The growth of the Japanese drug market has been spectacular. This country's per capita consumption was already the highest of all industrialized countries in 1975 and has continued to rise since then.

During the past decade, the pharmaceutical industry has undergone increasing consolidation. Domestic and international mergers, joint ventures, and strategic alliances proliferated in the global pharmaceutical industry in the 1980s. The main reason for the consolidation is the increase in R&D costs in recent years. Manufacturer's profits are also being squeezed by increasing pressure from national governments to contain health costs.

Of the top ten leading companies in R&D expenditures for 1996/97, five were U.S.-based, four were European, and one was a U.S.-Sweden combination. The average proportion of sales allocated to R&D by these companies was 16 percent. Novartis (formed by a merger of Ciba and Sandoz) of Switzerland had the largest R&D budget in the pharmaceutical industry. However, Roche of Germany had the highest R&D expenditure-to-sales ratio of 20 percent.

EVOLUTION OF THE GLOBAL INDUSTRY

Figure 1.1 illustrates the important milestones in the evolution of the global pharmaceutical industry.[1] One of the earliest milestones was the pre-World War II development and commercial marketing by the German chemical industry of a number of synthetically derived pharmaceutical products.

Many of the early chemical companies, such as those in Switzerland and Germany, found that their technology to make synthetic dyes was readily transferable to pharmaceuticals, resulting in the development and commercialization of a number of new pharmaceu-

FIGURE 1.1. Important Milestones in the Evolution of the Global Pharmaceutical Industry

1899	Discovery of aspirin
1906	Pure Food and Drug Act (United States)
1908	Discovery of Salversan (Germany)
1914	World War I
1931	FDA established (United States)
1935	Discovery of sulfa drugs
1939	World War II
1940	United States spends $3 million on penicillin research
1950-1960	Multinational expansion by U.S. firms
1962	Kefauver-Harris Amendment to the FDCA
1975	Revision of Japanese investment policies
1975-1985	Dramatic rise in biotech firms in the United States
1989	Mergers/acquisitions
1990-1995	Patents on approximately 200 products expired in the United States

Source: Adapted from USITC (1991).

tical products between 1908 and World War II. Advances in pharmaceutical production technology were also made during this time.

The Swiss industry had established facilities early in the United States, becoming one of the first to become truly multinational in an effort to compensate for their relatively small domestic market. After World War II, however, the U.S. industry rapidly expanded overseas. The pharmaceutical industry worldwide became truly global in scope after World War II. Several interrelated factors contributed to this trend. Significant advances in technology that led to the discovery of newer, more effective therapy took place in this period. Manufacturing know-how increased, enabling production of pharmaceuticals in huge quantities. Demand for medications increased the world over because of their greater effectiveness and availability. This was coupled with increased economic growth leading to greater purchasing power of consumers, helped by national health insurance systems in some countries.

In recent years internationalization of the pharmaceutical industry has been driven by a combination of reasons specific to the industry:

1. Development costs for a marketable new drug are very high and growing rapidly. These costs have to be spread over the widest possible market.
2. Product life cycles are fairly short, leading to a need to maximize global sales as quickly as possible.
3. The bulk of profits comes from patented products, again providing a motive to move overseas wherever patent protection can be obtained.

However, to better understand the tremendous changes taking place in the post-World War II period, three important eras are examined, namely: (a) 1940-1960, The Golden Era; (b) 1960-1980, Era of Regulation; and (c) 1980 to the present, Era of Consolidation (Agrawal, 1993).

1940-1960: The Golden Era

Several synthetic compounds were discovered in this period. The availability of a wide range of synthetic compounds and the advent of public health care systems, coupled with a surge in economic prosperity and political stability, created a tremendous growth in the international pharmaceutical market (Keller and Smith, 1969).

During this period, U.S. drug firms dramatically increased their investment abroad. Between 1950 and 1959, the total value of U.S. investment abroad rose from $12 billion to almost $30 billion. A prominent observer during this period dubbed this phenomenon of frenzied international expansion as the "gold rush" (Moskowitz, 1961).

The key factor in the early success of the American drug companies was their technological leadership. A number of important pharmacologic innovations in the United States, particularly in the antibiotic and corticosteroid fields, produced a virtual revolution in the pharmaceutical marketplace. Technological leadership coupled with adequate resources and a lack of organized competition enabled many of the larger American drug companies to secure important market positions. By 1960, the United States led in the drug export race, with Switzerland, Great Britain, West Germany, and France also in the race (*Chemical Engineering News*, 1961).

1960-1980: The Era of Regulation

This period was characterized by increasing public discontent with the industry, especially in the United States and Britain, leading to greater regulatory controls over the practices of drug firms. Cries of "unethical promotion," "excess profits," "soaring costs of drugs," and the like were commonly heard (*Chemical Engineering News*, 1961).

The thalidomide disaster[2] served as the catalyst for increased regulatory reforms being implemented (Smith, 1983). The United States passed the Kefauver-Harris amendment in 1961, which imposed serious regulatory controls over American-based companies. This amendment made pharmaceutical research a more expensive and time-consuming process by requiring substantial evidence of efficacy for approval of new drugs.

West Germany introduced new regulations concerning advertising of pharmaceuticals and related products during this period. Stringent governmental rules discouraged several smaller firms from venturing abroad in the 1960s and 1970s.

1980 to the Present: The Era of Consolidation

Domestic and international mergers, joint ventures, and strategic alliances proliferated in the global pharmaceutical industry in the

1980s. According to one study, approximately 131 firms announced acquisitions or strategic alliances in the first six months of 1990, compared with a total of 51 in 1989 and 56 in 1988 (USITC, 1991). In the past two decades, the traditional strengths of the pharmaceutical companies—patented products, pricing flexibility, and steady innovation—have begun to erode. Downward pressures on pharmaceutical sales and prices have continued as governments around the world try various means to tackle the problem of escalating health care costs. Competition from generics has led to further erosion of pharmaceutical profits for big name manufacturers. 1997 was the year when an icon of the modern pharmaceutical age, Glaxo-Wellcome's H2-antagonist, Zantac, finally faced competition in the United States and the United Kingdom. Bereft of patent protection, Zantac's U.S. sales fell by 55 percent in three months.

These developments have led companies to merge or enter into joint ventures with each other. The largest merger of all time took place in 1996 between the two Swiss giants Ciba and Sandoz, which merged to form a new health care company called Novartis. This trend of acquisitions and mergers is expected to continue in the future, in an attempt to reduce R&D costs, boost marketing revenues, and enable technology sharing.

DETERMINANTS OF COMPETITIVENESS IN THE GLOBAL PHARMACEUTICAL INDUSTRY

A study conducted by the U.S. International Trade Commission in 1991 on the global competitiveness of the U.S. pharmaceutical industry concluded that:

1. The competitiveness of the U.S. pharmaceutical industry, as well as those in other countries, depends largely on the ability of firms within the industry to develop innovative products, and innovation in turn depends on the ability to finance R&D.
2. Government policies, both domestic and foreign, have a more significant effect on the level of industry innovation than many of the other factors studied (USITC, 1991).

The USITC study concluded that the U.S. pharmaceutical industry maintained a high degree of competitiveness from 1980 to 1990, compared with the industries in Western Europe and Japan. The study found that the U.S. industry was a leader in innovation from 1975 to 1989, developing the majority of the globally successful products introduced during this time period.

This is in contrast to the conclusions published in the report of a study done by the National Academy of Sciences (NAE, 1983) to assess the competitive position of the U.S. pharmaceutical industry in the world economy. The study found a declining trend in the U.S. share of R&D expenditures and drugs entering clinical trials, and predicted further decline in U.S. shares of pharmaceutical introductions, sales, and exports.

Further, more recent data indicates that Japanese companies may be catching on. For example, for the years 1982 to 1993, Japan introduced 158 new chemical entities, whereas the United States introduced 123 new chemical entities in the same period (author's estimates, *Scrip Magazine*—various issues). Although these NCEs do not represent globally successful NCEs[3] in which the United States is still a leader, the data should still be a cause for concern.

Figure 1.2 illustrates the pattern of NCE introduction from 1961 to 1990 by the United States, Western Europe, and Japan. The number of NCEs originating from the United States and Western

FIGURE 1.2. NCE Introductions by the United States, Western Europe, and Japan

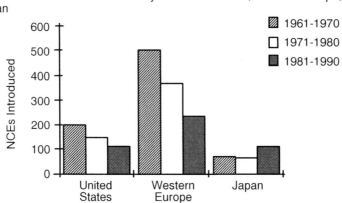

Source: Author's estimates based on various sources.

Europe show a declining trend, whereas the number of NCEs originating from Japan show an upward trend for the past decade.

SUMMARY

The global pharmaceutical industry is highly multinational and research intensive. It is dominated by companies from the United States, Western Europe, and Japan. Over the years, the industry has faced increasing regulatory pressures from national governments and in the recent past has been characterized by mergers and strategic alliance formation. The industry combines a unique blend of scientific knowledge, manufacturing skills, and marketing tactics. Competitiveness in the global industry depends on ability to innovate (develop new drugs) and overcome market and regulatory barriers of varying country markets.

Chapter 2

National Environment
and Global Competition

This chapter reviews the theoretical, conceptual, and empirical
literature on the effect of national environmental factors on the
global competitiveness of any industry. Three perspectives are examined: (1) national competitiveness—theoretical and conceptual
perspectives, (2) competitiveness in the global pharmaceutical industry, and (3) global strategic perspectives.

NATIONAL COMPETITIVENESS—
THEORETICAL AND CONCEPTUAL PERSPECTIVES

National competitiveness has become one of the central pre-
occupations of government and industry in every nation, especially
in the United States. The competitiveness of the U.S. economy in
the global market became a growing concern during the 1980s, due
to sustained deterioration in the U.S. trade deficit. The loss of
market share in products such as microelectronics, an industry
many thought invulnerable to foreign competition, began to raise
questions regarding the overall international competitiveness of the
U.S. economy. Yet for all the discussion, debate, and writing on the
topic, there is still no persuasive theory to explain national competitiveness (Porter, 1990).

Definition of National Competitiveness

An accepted definition of the term "competitiveness" is lacking.
Some see national competitiveness as a macroeconomic phenomenon,

driven by variables such as exchange rates, interest rates, and government deficits. Others argue that competitiveness is a function of cheap and abundant labor. Another popular explanation for national competitiveness focuses on differences in management practices, including management-labor relations. Porter (1990) identifies productivity as the major determinant of a nation's competitiveness. According to the President's Commission on Industrial Competitiveness,

> competitiveness is the degree to which a nation can, under free and fair market conditions, produce goods and services that meet the test of international markets while simultaneously maintaining or expanding the real incomes of its citizens. (Commission on Industrial Competitiveness, 1985)

The lack of clarity on the definition of national competitiveness is due in part to the fact that competitiveness is a multidimensional concept that cannot be reduced to a single variable or indicator. A second difficulty arises from the fact that it is difficult to consider indicators of competitive position separately, without reference to underlying causal variables (Hatzichronoglou, 1991).

Although it is appropriate to consider international competitiveness at the national level, it has a different meaning when applied at the industry or individual firm level. For example, at the sectoral level, competitiveness may be defined as the ability of an industry or firm to sustain and/or expand its market position. Competitiveness at the national sectoral levels are intertwined, however, because it depends on the competitive strength of firms and/or industries to generate productivity levels needed to support high wages and hence higher standards of living in the economy. Similarly, sector competitiveness depends on appropriate policy at the national level that would, for example, provide a framework for the promotion of high levels of skill through education and maintenance and/or development of infrastructure. Bruce Scott of the Harvard Business School has defined national competitiveness as:

> a nation state's ability to produce, distribute and service goods in the international economy in competition with goods and services produced by other countries, and to do so in a way that earns a rising standard of living. (Scott and Lodge, 1985)

There are three critical aspects to this definition. First, it is *trade based*, that is, the export performance of a nation is considered relative to that of others. Second, it is a *performance based* concept, that is, the ability of a nation to earn a higher standard of living by production and marketing skills, rather than by international borrowings. Third, it is a *dynamic* concept, as it evaluates the manner in which a nation seeks to increase and distribute its welfare over time, given its international and domestic commitments.

Theory of Comparative Advantage

This theory, also referred to as the classical theory, explains the success of nations in particular industries based on so-called factors of production such as land, labor, and natural resources. Nations gain factor-based comparative advantage in industries that make intensive use of the factors they possess in abundance. Classical theory, however, has been overshadowed in advanced industries and economies by the globalization of competition and the power of technology.

The Technology Factor Theory

Although there may be little agreement on the definition of competitiveness, there is general consensus in the more recent literature that national competitiveness depends on much more than the cost of production and prices of output. Technology is increasingly recognized as the most important determinant to achieving competitive advantage in the global economy (Niosi, 1991; Scott and Lodge, 1985; Porter, 1990; Ernst and O'Connor, 1989). Recent studies on international competitiveness emphasize the central role played by technology in determining the world market share (Davis, 1991; Dosi and Soete, 1991; Scott and Lodge, 1985; Ernst and O'Connor, 1989; Porter, 1990).

The role of technology and innovation in the economic growth of a nation has been emphasized by industrial economists since the time of Schumpeter. Posner (1961), Gomulka (1971), and Cornwall (1976) developed this approach into what they referred to as the technology gap theory.

The technology gap theorists relate the technological level of a country to its *level of innovative activity.* A high level of innovative activity means a high share of new goods in output and an extensive use of new techniques in production. Because new goods command high prices and new techniques imply high productivity, it follows that countries with a comparatively higher level of innovative activities also tend to have a higher level of value added per worker, or gross domestic product (GDP) per capita, than other countries. According to Louis Emmerij, President of OECD:

> Today, oligopolistic competition and strategic interaction, rather than the "invisible hand" of market forces, condition comparative advantage and the international division of labor. The introduction of new technologies plays an important role in this process. Firms as much as nations are striving to utilize technology as an instrument of global competition. (Ernst and O'Connor, 1989, p. 8)

When one looks at any national economy, there are striking differences in competitive success among a nation's industries. International advantage is often concentrated in particular industry segments. In many industries and segments of industries, the competitors with true international competitive advantage are based in only a few nations.

Porter's study (1990) examined high-technology industries in ten important trading nations to investigate why nations gain competitive advantage in particular industries and the implications for company strategy and national economies. The study found that a nation's competitiveness in a particular industry depends on its capacity to innovate and upgrade. Companies from such nations gain advantage against the world's best competitors because of pressure and challenge. They benefit from having strong domestic rivals, aggressive home-based suppliers, and demanding local customers.

Four broad attributes of a nation contribute to innovation and subsequent national competitiveness, both individually and as a system. These attributes are: factor conditions (labor, infrastructure, etc.); demand conditions (nature of home-market demand); related and supporting industries; and firm strategy, structure, and rivalry.

In addition, differences in national values, economic structures, institutions, and histories all contribute to competitive success.

The study also concluded that the proper role of government is as a catalyst and a challenger; to encourage—or even push—companies to raise their aspirations and move to higher levels of competitive performance. Government policies that succeed are those that create an environment in which companies can gain competitive advantage.

The literature on international technology transfer also provides some insights on competitiveness in the global economy (Robinson, 1991). Competitiveness in high-technology industries depends on: (a) supply of technology, (b) demand for technology, and (c) intermediaries and linking mechanisms.

The Role of Government and Public Policy

The role of government and public policy in a nation's effort to achieve international competitiveness has been a subject of much debate. Three major policy recommendations have been offered in the literature: (1) the activist industrial policy perspective, (2) the managed trade perspective, and (3) the neoclassical or liberal economics perspective.

Activist Industrial Policy Perspective

The advocates of industrial policies in the early 1980s recommended an active government role to enable all industries within an advanced economy to shift production toward higher value-added and more competitive outputs (Wachter and Wachter, 1982; Magaziner and Reich, 1982; Adams and Klein, 1982; Johnson, 1984). For declining industries, for example, proponents of the activist industrial policies recommend that agreements between the United States and governments of other advanced nations should be worked out to ease adjustment of less competitive firms by granting subsidies as well as protection from imports for a limited period, as needed. For emerging businesses with highly skilled employees and characterized by rapid technological change, the U.S. government should provide subsidies, loan guarantees, and tax benefits to lure them to locate at home rather than abroad.

The Managed Trade Perspective

Managed trade can be broadly defined as trade that is controlled, directed, or administered by government policies and conducted by either bilateral or multilateral agreements (USITC, 1991). The proponents of managed trade recommend some form of government involvement in high-technology industries (Reich, 1983; Tyson, 1990; Goldstein and Krasner, 1984). They suggest that the fate of these industries cannot be left solely to market forces, particularly in the presence of activist government intervention abroad. They recommend active intervention in the form of export subsidies and import restrictions. Both the activist industrial policy and managed trade proponents use Japanese trade performance to support their views, because they consider Japan's success a case study of how a country can realize its trade-related goals through extensive but carefully planned protectionism.

Liberal Economics Perspective

The proponents of the liberal or neoclassical perspective reject the activist industrial and managed trade policy recommendations for enhancing the U.S. economy's international competitiveness (Commission on Industrial Competitiveness, 1985; Dixit, 1986; Hatsopoulos, Krugman, and Summers, 1988; Porter, 1990; Landau, 1990). They argue that pursuing such a strategic trade policy would require vast, unknown amounts of information about the economy and externalities associated with interventionist policy. Also, most economists believe that such policies could result in raised costs for other sectors within the economy and in trade wars. The liberal economics view of promoting the U.S. economy's international competitiveness and increasing the standard of living is perhaps the most accepted view in the economics literature.

For example, Porter (1990) recommends the following government initiatives for national competitiveness: maintain a strong antitrust policy to foster domestic competition; maintain an open trade policy and avoid devaluation to boost exports; create incentives for higher savings and allow interest rates to fall to encourage investment and longer time horizons on R&D projects; and fund university research centers to rejuvenate national R&D.

Industrial Innovation and Public Policy

Since innovation drives technological growth and therefore industrial competitiveness, it is important to look at the effect regulation can have on industrial innovation processes.

More studies have been done on the factors endogenous to the
firm in attempting to explain innovative success or failure; that is,
they have considered the innovation process more or less exclusively from the point of view of what managers have—or have
not—done and generally neglected external factors such as the role
of government (Rothwell and Zegveld, 1981). The studies that have
examined the impact of regulation on industrial innovation processes are reviewed below.

Perhaps more has been written about the effects of regulation on the
rate of innovation in pharmaceuticals than in any other single sector of
the industry (Hauptman and Roberts, 1987; Young, 1982; Grabowski
and Vernon, 1976; Grabowski, Vernon, and Thomas, 1978; Hansen,
1979; Peltzman, DiRaddo, and Fringeri, 1980; Peltzman, May, and
Trimble, 1982; Wiggins, 1981, 1983; Brownlee, 1979; Clymer, 1970,
1975; Cooper, 1969, 1976; Jaffe, 1976; Lasagna, 1969; Lasagna and
Wardell, 1975; Mitchell and Link, 1976; Sarett, 1974; Schankerman,
1976; Schwartzman, 1976; Wardell, 1973, 1974).

Much that has been written has focused on the impact of the 1962
Kefauver-Harris Amendments to the U.S. Food, Drug, and Cosmet-
ics Act.[1] Most analyses of the effects of regulation on innovation in
the U.S. drug industry have treated the 1962 amendments as a
watershed. According to Peltzman (1973), for example, the 1962
amendments significantly reduced the flow of New Chemical
Entities (NCEs) into the market. Furthermore, all the observed
differences between the pre- and post-1963 NCE flows could be
attributed to the 1962 amendments.

A study done by Steward (1977) of the new pharmaceutical
products and new chemicals introduced in the United States between 1948 and 1975 demonstrated a marked decrease in both
quantities during the 1960s. However, when comparable data for
the United Kingdom was used, it also indicated a decline in total
pharmaceutical products and in new chemical entities beginning
around 1960. Thus, it would appear that the Kefauver-Harris

Amendments were not the only factor causing a decline in pharmaceutical innovations in the United States, but that the decline was part of a broader, underlying phenomenon that was operating worldwide. Comparison of the U.S. and UK data does show, however, that the *rate* of decline was very much sharper in the United States than in the United Kingdom, which might be taken to indicate the added impact in the United States of the 1962 amendments.

However, it is not only the *quantity* of new drugs which is important, but also their *quality*, that is, their therapeutic significance. Using data for the years 1950 to 1973, Steward (1977) examined the annual approval of NCEs by degree of therapeutic importance.[2] It was found that while there was a general downward trend for drugs offering modest gain and little or no gain, the 1962 amendments had little impact on the rate of introduction of drugs offering an important gain. However, a marked decrease in new introductions for all three classes of drugs was found to have occurred between 1966 and 1969. This might represent the true impact of the 1962 amendments, taking into account the lead times inherent in new drug development.

Another effect of regulation on innovation of pharmaceuticals is in delaying the market launch of new products and processes through lengthening approval times. There is also evidence to suggest that because of the greater strictness of regulation in the United States, important new drugs are sometimes marketed there many years after their acceptance in other countries. For example, in 1989, 18 of the 23 new products approved for marketing in the United States had received their first marketing approval in countries other than the United States. From 1984 to 1988, 88 of the 113 products introduced in the United States were first approved in a foreign country (PMA, 1989).

Later in this chapter, additional regulatory effects such as patent laws, pricing policies, and product liability laws on pharmaceutical innovation are discussed.

COMPETITIVENESS IN THE GLOBAL PHARMACEUTICAL INDUSTRY

Empirical analysis of competitiveness in the global pharmaceutical industry has concentrated primarily on factors influencing the supply of ethical pharmaceutical products (factors affecting innovation). Further, much of the analysis is related to or in response to the debate regarding the effects of regulatory measures and other government policies on the industry. For the most part, research has focused on the activities of U.S. firms in the U.S. market. Empirical analysis of the U.S. industry's competitive position in the international market is relatively limited.

Role of Regulation, R&D, and Innovation

Research is the foundation of competitive strength for modern pharmaceutical firms. Growth in sales and profits for major drug companies are derived from successful new products discovered and developed through industry research efforts. Pharmaceutical research may be divided into four phases:

1. *Basic research:* advancement of basic pharmacological knowledge. This is the only phase not directly regulated by the government, although government regulation has a substantial indirect influence.
2. *Discovery effort:* the synthesis of active substances and the establishment of biological effect.
3. *Applied research:* the extensive biological (animal) and clinical (human) testing of substances to determine pharmacological activity and risk of adverse effects.
4. *Development:* the determination of dosage form, the development of manufacturing processes, and the production of drug product.

Because investment in R&D is one of the most important criteria for success in the pharmaceutical industry, and because regulation is one of the most common factors affecting R&D investment decisions of firms, most empirical studies have concentrated on the effect of regulation on R&D as mentioned previously.

The most recent study to date was done by the U.S. International Trade Commission (USITC, 1991). This study was done to assess the competitive position of the U.S. pharmaceutical industry in the global economy.

This study used two data sets. The first data set consisted of various annual economic, demographic, and health-related measures from 1983 to 1988 for seven countries who had competitive pharmaceutical industries. These were: France, Germany, Italy, Japan, Spain, the United Kingdom, and the United States. This data set was used to do a country-level analysis.

The second data set comprised various measures relating to R&D, firm size, and sales for a sample of pharmaceutical firms from the United States, Western Europe, and Japan. A total of twenty-nine firms were used. This data set was used to do a regional comparison at the firm level. The analysis consisted of a number of regression estimates. The main findings of the study were:

1. A growing national economy provides an important underlying base for the pharmaceutical industry. Growth in national income, growth in GDP/per capita, and a higher life expectancy were used as indicators of a growing economy.
2. National research efforts help foster the discovery of innovative NCEs, and relatively higher prices for pharmaceuticals partially explain the larger number of NCEs introduced into a country.
3. Higher levels of R&D expenditures and R&D employees are important for global market share and productivity.

Grabowski (1989) examined the competitiveness of the U.S. pharmaceutical industry with respect to indicators such as: (1) number of new products under development in 1986 by corporate nationality; (2) new product introductions by corporate nationality from 1961 to 1986; (3) number of global NCEs by nationality of originating firm from 1970 to 1983; and (4) worldwide sales by corporate nationality for 1980, 1984, and 1986. The countries for which the above data was compared were the United States, Japan, West Germany, France, Italy, Switzerland, and the United Kingdom.

However, no statistical tests were conducted. The raw data were simply examined for major trends in order to draw conclusions. Grabowski concluded that the U.S. industry is currently the leader in worldwide sales, R&D activity, and new drug candidates under development. The U.S. industry was also found to be significantly more responsible for commercially important new drugs and global NCEs.

Grabowski also cautioned that foreign competitors, particularly Japan, could provide a strong challenge to U.S. leadership in pharmaceuticals over the next few decades. The European pharmaceutical industries were found to have a generally declining position in the 1980s. This was attributed to control on drug prices in their domestic markets. Grabowski concludes by saying that current U.S. policies in the health sector are increasingly driven by priorities that could result in a less favorable economic environment for new product introductions.

The National Academy of Engineering conducted a study to evaluate the competitive status of the U.S. pharmaceutical industry in the international market (NAE, 1983). The study used six indicators to measure competitiveness: research effort, innovative output, production, sales, market structure, and international trade. Data for the United States, Western Europe, and Japan were compared. The study found a decline in U.S.-based drug production as a percentage of world drug production, and a decline in the U.S. share of world pharmaceutical R&D. A combination of factors was blamed for the decline: foreign nontariff barriers, U.S. FDA regulations, patent laws, product liability laws, antitrust policies, and R&D tax incentives.

The NAE study concluded that although the U.S. industry was likely to remain a significant force in the international market, decreases in various measures of industrial performance relative to other major international pharmaceutical producers suggested that the industry would lose its dominant position.

In a follow-up study by the U.S. Department of Commerce's International Trade Administration (ITA, 1984), it was concluded that the United States was and would continue to be internationally competitive. However, the study identified a number of policy issues that could affect the global position of the industry. It concluded that U.S. companies were likely to be at a disadvantage because of the significantly longer U.S. regulatory review periods.

Thomas (1989) compared the performance of the U.S. industry to that of other countries' industries using a ten-nation sample. He concluded that firms competing successfully in the international market do so by developing innovative new drugs that can be successfully marketed in most major country markets. He suggested that a critical factor contributing to a company's ability to compete successfully in the international market is the degree of competition in the company's home market. Three factors contribute to competitive home country markets: rigorous quality restrictions on market access, high levels of publicly funded biomedical research, and unregulated domestic prices.

A report issued by the Council on Competitiveness (1991) emphasizes that factors such as science education, funding for R&D, and relative freedom from price control are important to the continued competitiveness of the U.S. industry. Table 2.1 presents an overview of the studies on global pharmaceutical competitiveness.

TABLE 2.1. Overview of Studies on Global Pharmaceutical Competitiveness

Study	(a) Factors examined (b) Countries/Regions	Determinants of Competitiveness
USITC (1991)	(a) Economic, demographic, and social factors; R&D measures; firm size; and sales. (b) France, Germany, Italy, Japan, Spain, United Kingdom, and United States.	Innovation, growing economy, R&D incentives, low price control, R&D investment.
Grabowski (1989)	(a) Number of drugs under development; NCE introductions; global NCEs developed; global sales. (b) United States, Japan, Germany, France, Italy, Switzerland, and United Kingdom.	Innovation, R&D investment, commercial potential of NCE.
NAE (1983)	(a) Research investment; innovative output; production; sales; market structure; and trade balance. (b) United States, Japan, and Western Europe.	Regulatory conditions: FDA regulations, patent laws, product liability laws, antitrust policies, and R&D tax incentives.
ITA (1984)	(a) Sales; production; employment; productivity; R&D; and profitability data. (b) Industrialized countries.	Innovation, productivity of R&D, regulatory approval time, quality of NCE.
Thomas (1989)	(a) Various regulatory and market-related factors. (b) Industrialized countries.	Innovation, competitive markets, stringent quality regulations, high research funding, and unregulated domestic prices.
Council on Competitiveness (1991)	(a) Various regulatory and economic factors. (b) Industrialized countries.	Science education, R&D funding, and freedom from price control.

Pharmaceutical Diffusion and Competitiveness

As mentioned earlier, most conceptual and empirical work on competitiveness issues in the pharmaceutical industry has concentrated on supply factors, that is, factors that influence the extent and rate of pharmaceutical innovation.

However, as recently pointed out in the report by the U.S. International Trade Commission, it is equally important to look at factors that affect the intercountry diffusion of new pharmaceutical products, that is, factors affecting demand for pharmaceutical innovations across national markets. Knowledge of such factors provides the firm with a competitive advantage with respect to choosing markets more strategically for introduction of pharmaceutical innovations. It is also important from a public policy perspective to examine factors that delay market introduction of therapeutically significant drug innovations.

According to Redwood (1988), the ability to both innovate and market new drugs is crucial for global competitiveness and "one without the other is hardly a tenable proposition for survival in the upper reaches of the ethical sector of the pharmaceutical industry" (p. 72).

Only a handful of empirical studies have examined the factors affecting diffusion of pharmaceutical innovations in the international context. These few, with the exception of Parker's study (Parker, 1984), have focused on the effect of regulatory conditions on the international diffusion of new drugs.

Grabowski and Vernon (1977) analyzed the introduction of U.S.-discovered drugs into the United Kingdom from 1960 to 1972, to see the effect of the Kefauver-Harris Amendment on U.S. firms' strategy for foreign NCE introductions. A dramatic shift was found to have occurred as a result of the amendment. During the early 1960s, U.S. firms introduced a majority of the new drugs into the United Kingdom *only* after first introducing them into the United States. For the period 1972 to 1974, however, more than two-thirds of U.S.-discovered NCEs were first introduced into the United Kingdom instead of the United States.

Grabowski (1980) found a lag in foreign-discovered NCE introductions into the United States with respect to Europe. More seriously, the lag with Europe was not confined to drugs with little or modest therapeutic gain, but also included drugs that the FDA itself ranked as significant therapeutic advances. He considered regulatory changes the major factor contributing to the lag. Lag of foreign-discovered NCEs was especially significant because foreign-discovered NCEs accounted for one-half of the drugs rated therapeutically significant by the FDA during the period analyzed (1968 to 1973). These medically significant drugs of foreign origin were all introduced into the United States with very long time lags—three to six years after they were introduced into the United Kingdom.

LaFrancis-Popper and Nason (1994) examined the effect of various regulatory conditions using NCE introduction data over a twenty-year period, 1970 to 1989. The countries for which the data were collected were France, Germany, the United Kingdom, Italy, Japan, and the United States. The regulatory aspects that were examined for their effect on extent and timing of NCE introductions were: generic substitution, national health insurance plans, national formulary system, acceptance of foreign clinical testing, patent protection, compulsory out-licensing, and R&D pricing incentives.

Both generic substitution policies and the presence of national health plans seemed to increase diffusion lags. Compulsory out-licensing did not seem to affect number of product introductions, but it significantly increased the time taken for products to reach the market. Acceptance of foreign clinical data was associated with a shorter time lag to introduction, as were R&D pricing incentives. Market size was found to be positively related to number of product introductions but did not influence time lag for introduction.

The most comprehensive study to date on international diffusion of pharmaceuticals is the study by Parker (1984). Parker used a sample of eighteen countries comprising nine industrialized and nine developing countries. The time frame used in the study was from 1954 to 1978. A total of 192 brand-name pharmaceuticals were included in the analysis. The arrival time lag or diffusion lag was the dependent variable. This was measured as the time between marketing of the drug for the first time in a country and its subsequent marketing elsewhere. The independent variables examined were: regulatory tightness of country, therapeutic importance of drug, market attractiveness, and type of country.

Countries with the toughest regulatory environments had the lowest mean arrival time lags. Parker attributed this surprising result to the relationship between market size and regulatory environment. The countries with the stringent regulatory environments were also the ones with the large market size. Therefore countries with a larger market size seemed to attract products earlier than those with a smaller market size in spite of the regulatory climate. Mean arrival time lags were shorter for more important drugs than for less important drugs, but the relationship was not significant. With respect to type of country, drug introductions were fewer among the less developed economies, as well as having higher mean arrival time lags. Table 2.2 presents an overview of the studies on global pharmaceutical diffusion.

TABLE 2.2. Overview of Studies on Global Pharmaceutical Diffusion

Study	(a) Factors examined (b) Countries/Regions	Findings
Grabowski and Vernon (1977)	(a) Regulatory approval time. (b) United States and United Kingdom.	Diffusion lag in the United States due to longer approval times.
Grabowski (1980)	(a) Regulatory approval time; therapeutic importance of NCE. (b) United States and Europe.	Diffusion lag in the United States due to longer approval time.
LaFrancis-Popper and Nason (1994)	(a) Regulatory aspects; market size. (b) France, Germany, United Kingdom, Italy, Japan, and United States.	Regulatory aspects affect rate and extent of diffusion.
Parker (1984)	(a) Regulation; therapeutic importance of NCE; market size; type of country. (b) Nine industrialized and nine developing countries.	Regulation and market size interact to affect diffusion; diffusion is faster for more important NCEs; and developing countries have longer diffusion lags.

Supply and Demand Factors
in Pharmaceutical Competitiveness

Figure 2.1 illustrates the various supply and demand factors affecting competitiveness in the global pharmaceutical industry. As shown in the figure, the demand for ethical pharmaceuticals is determined by demographic and socioeconomic factors, such as age of the population, diet, or access to health care, etc. Government policies and programs such as cost-containment, degree of health-care financing, and support for health-related education may also affect the demand for drugs, directly or indirectly.

An important factor affecting the supply of ethical pharmaceuticals is R&D activity, that is, the level and productivity of R&D spending. Such activity requires sufficiently high profits, the ability to secure external financing, or both. Government actions ranging from macroeconomic policies, treatment of product liability, tax policy, and regulatory controls exert indirect and direct effects (positive and negative) on the ability of firms and the industry as a whole to produce pharmaceuticals.

A discussion of the demographic, social, economic, political, legal, and market-related characteristics that affect the international supply and demand for pharmaceutical innovations follows.

Demographic Environment and Competitiveness

National differences in population density, life expectancy, birth rate, death rate, composition, distribution, and so on create variations in market conditions that offer opportunities as well as threats. They also influence supply and demand.

The larger the market potential for pharmaceuticals in a particular country, the greater will be the incentive for the firms in that country to innovate and introduce new products. A key demographic factor affecting market potential for ethical pharmaceuticals is the proportion of the elderly in the population. Projections show that this population in many industrialized countries is growing rapidly.

The frequency of drug consumption is rising most rapidly in markets where the population is aging. For example, data for Germany show that roughly 55 percent of the population over age forty-four takes drugs at least once a week, but only 15 percent of

FIGURE 2.1. Determination of Global Market Share in the Pharmaceutical Industry

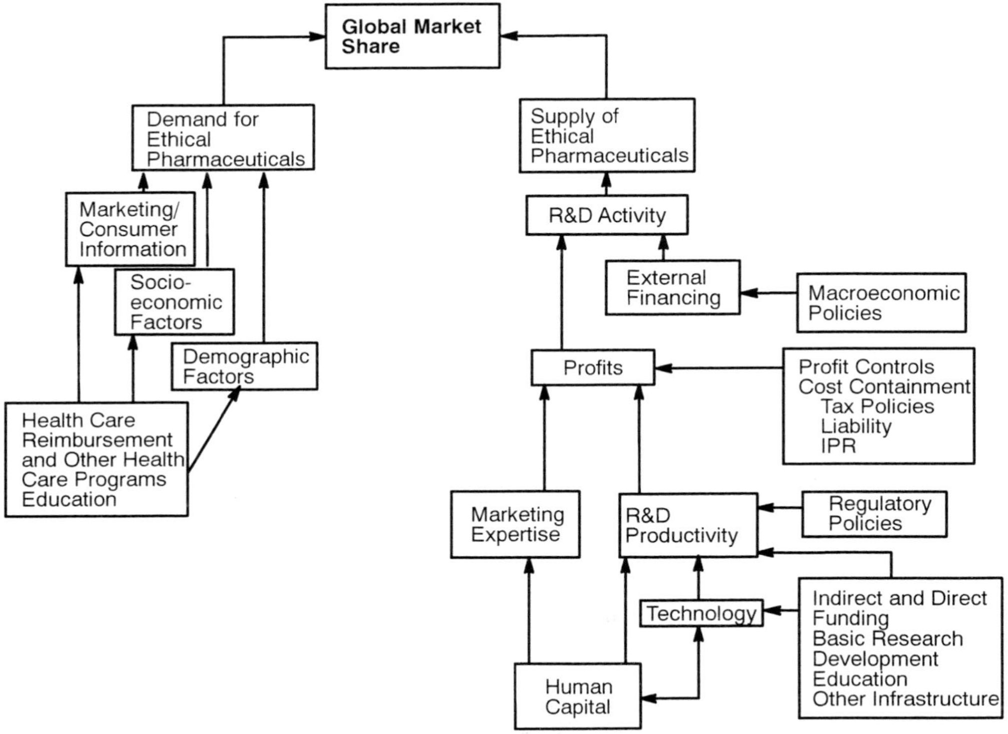

Source: USITC (1991).

those between fourteen and forty-four years of age consume drugs this frequently (Ballance, Pogany, and Forstner, 1992). Moreover, the types of drugs required by individuals under forty-five years of age are different from those purchased by the elderly. They consist mainly of painkillers, cough and cold preparations, and digestives. These are frequently generics and are less expensive than other drug types.

One-sixth of all Germans will be over sixty-five by the year 2000, and by 2010 half the country's population will be fifty years of age or older. In contrast, in a developing country such as India only 25 percent of the population will be fifty or older by 2010 (Redwood, 1988).

Social Environment and Competitiveness

These factors include the health care systems of the country—private and public, dispensing practices of physicians, nature of consumer demand for pharmaceuticals, and so on. The types of national health care systems in industrialized and developing countries differ greatly, and their effects on the pattern of pharmaceutical consumption are equally disparate.

Governments in industrialized countries established very generous systems of health care during periods when national income was rising and the proportion of old people in the population was comparatively small. The public sector in most industrialized countries accounts for more than half of all drug expenditures. The only exceptions are Canada and the United States; in both of these countries, a large portion of pharmaceutical expenditures is covered by private medical insurance or involves direct payments by patients (Ballance, Pogany, and Forstner, 1992).

Systems of public health care are a less significant determinant of consumption in the developing countries. The main reason is the small proportion of total income available for this purpose. Public expenditures on health care in most developing countries account for between 1 and 2 percent of gross national product (GNP), while in the industrialized countries the figure is much higher, typically between 6 and 8 percent. As much as two-thirds of the drugs purchased by patients in poor and medium-income developing countries are paid for privately (Redwood, 1988, pp. 254-256).

Both the supply and demand for pharmaceutical innovations will be affected by the nature of the public health systems. The greater the public health expenditure in a country, the greater will be the demand (hence diffusion) for new drugs as well as the investments in the innovation process to generate NCEs due to the larger size of the market.

Several industrialized countries are now being forced to cut back on their health care programs, and pharmaceuticals are a favorite target. Reasons for the cutbacks include the rising costs of caring for an aging population, the introduction of new and more expensive drugs, and a general tightening of federal budgets. Because a large portion of the total spending on drugs is paid for through public funds, the change in policy is having a dramatic effect on consumption. The steps taken by policymakers include the introduction of stricter policy controls, the withdrawal of reimbursements from selected products, and increases in patient contributions to the cost of drugs.

Doctors in several industrialized countries are now coming under pressure to prescribe more economically and to use generic substitutes. This tactic is most popular in the United States where generics accounted for 29 percent of all the country's drug sales in 1988. The same is not the case in Western Europe. The slow rate of acceptance is partly due to opposition from industry representatives and from the medical profession. Both groups have vigorously resisted legislation to promote generic substitution.

Economic Environment and Competitiveness

These factors include the overall level of development of the originating countries, per capita income and distribution, disposable income, expenditure patterns, and so on. The pharmaceutical industry is highly research oriented and development of new ethical pharmaceuticals runs into millions of dollars.

Developed-country firms based in a growing or robust economy are the only ones that can afford such costly investment. For example, Western European and American drug companies have accounted for nearly 80 percent of all NMEs (new molecular entities) launched from 1961 to 1990 (USITC, 1991).

The economic attractiveness of markets is likely to have a significant influence on the rate of intercountry spread of drugs. Wealthy countries with large markets for pharmaceuticals may exert a strong commercial pull and attract foreign-developed drugs earlier than poorer nations with less purchasing power.

For example, the U.S. pharmaceutical industry has invested extensively throughout the world. However, investment by the U.S. pharmaceutical industry in the developed nations accounted for about 75 percent of the total investment in 1986, with developing countries accounting for only 25 percent. The major markets for U.S. drug exports in 1989 were Japan (21 percent of total), Germany (10 percent), Canada (8 percent), and Italy (6 percent). The top seven pharmaceutical markets in the world accounted for 77 percent of the world pharmaceutical sales in 1989. These countries were France, Germany, Italy, Japan, Spain, the United Kingdom, and the United States. Thus the extent of diffusion is clearly affected by market attractiveness (U.S. Department of Commerce, 1989).

More than 70 percent of all pharmaceuticals are sold in developed market economies. The developing countries account for less than a fifth, with the remainder being consumed in East European countries and the former USSR (Ballance, Pogany, and Forstner, 1992; see Figure 2.2). Japan reports the largest share of per capita income spent on pharmaceuticals (1.62 percent in 1990)—almost twice the level in North America and some parts of Western Europe. No similar increases have occurred in developing countries. In fact, the share of per capita GDP spent on pharmaceuticals has actually declined in many of the poorer countries.

Political Environment and Competitiveness

Factors such as political stability and continuity, ideological orientation, government involvement in business, attitudes toward MNCs, national economic and developmental priorities, and so on, will affect a firm's ability and propensity to invest in R&D and thus its supply of innovative pharmaceutical products (Thorelli, 1990; Toyne and Walters, 1993). The industrialized countries are the most stable politically and emphasize basic research priorities. Firms from such countries are therefore likely to invest heavily in R&D and produce more new chemical entities.

FIGURE 2.2. World Consumption of Pharmaceuticals, 1992

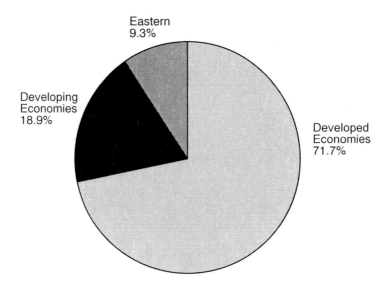

Source: Ballance, Pogany, and Forstner, 1992.

Political factors will also affect a firm's decision to introduce a new product in a particular country (Thorelli, 1990; Toyne and Walters, 1993). The greater the number of destination countries with high political instability, high government involvement in business, high hostility of the government toward foreign firms or MNCs, and/or differing ideologies of the governments, the lower will be the extent and rate of global diffusion of the product. For example, the pharmaceutical market share held by domestic firms in the former Soviet Union in 1985 was 100 percent with zero percent foreign involvement. In comparison, market share by domestic firms in Canada was only 18 percent in 1985, reflecting the high investment by foreign firms in Canada (Pradhan, 1983).

Legal Environment and Competitiveness

Government policies, whether domestic or international, can have a significant impact on both the rate and extent of innovation in a country's industry as well as on rate and extent of diffusion of NCEs into the country, given the nature of the industry.

These government policies include regulatory approval procedures, pricing policies, cost-containment efforts, patent law and intellectual property rights, product liability laws, and tariff-related matters such as granting of duty suspensions. Figure 2.3 illustrates the entire drug development cycle starting from basic research to market approval to patent expiry and finally reinvestment in the research process. As seen in the figure, much of the area of maximum risk is also that of maximum intervention by regulatory authorities, reaching a financial climax when it comes to pricing and social security reimbursement.

As has been described in the previous sections, the role of regulation, in particular the effect of changes in the U.S. regulatory procedure for market approval of NCEs, has been the subject of analysis in a majority of the studies on pharmaceutical innovation and diffusion. The empirical studies examining this issue have been discussed previously; thus the following section will only focus on the regulatory approval procedures of other countries in comparison to the United States. Also, other aspects of regulation mentioned previously that affect the supply and demand for innovation are discussed below.

Regulatory approval for new drugs. Approval varies by country. Generally under the FDCA, a new drug may not be commercially marketed in the United States unless it has been approved as safe and effective by the FDA. The average FDA review time for the twenty new drugs approved in the United States in 1988 was about thirty-one months, compared with an average of approximately fifteen months for foreign review of those of the twenty products that were first approved overseas (PMA, 1989). The drug development process from discovery to FDA approval takes approximately ten years. Any delays in the development and marketing approval process shortens a product's effective patent life, reducing the period in which a company can recoup its R&D expenditures.

FIGURE 2.3. Risks in Pharmaceutical R&D

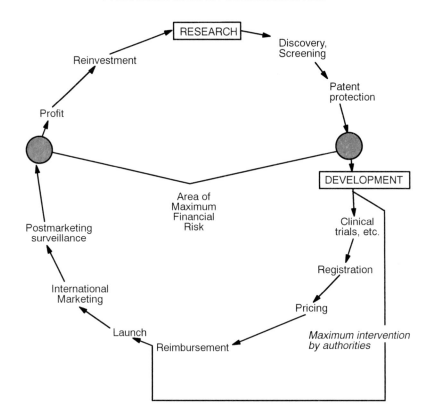

Source: Adapted from Redwood (1991).

Regulatory approval procedures of different countries affect perceived market attractiveness and thus affect the decision of a firm with respect to the choice of country for first launch of a new product. Industry sources state that a perceived differential in approval times prompts many companies to seek market approvals overseas first. For example, in 1989, eighteen of the twenty-three products approved in the United States had received their first marketing approval in countries other than the United States. From

1984 through 1988, 88 of the 113 products introduced in the United States were first approved in a foreign country (PMA, 1989).

Drug approval regulations in Japan also inhibit diffusion of drugs into that country. Foreign firms in Japan were prohibited from applying on their own for the first step of drug approval, that is, the demonstration of efficacy and safety review, and clinical trials had to be conducted in Japan on native citizens. Both policies remained in effect until the mid-1980s, when discussions with the United States in bilateral trade negotiations resulted in changes that allowed foreign firms to apply directly and permitted the submission of the results of foreign clinical trials. However, incompatibility of the data is still an issue in many areas. Some human clinical studies must still be performed in Japan, to Japanese standards, resulting in duplication of efforts for foreign firms (*Medical Marketing,* 1990).

Efforts have been made for international harmonization of approval procedures in the recent years. In 1991, the International Conference on the Harmonization of Technical Requirements for Registration of Pharmaceuticals was held in Brussels. The objective of the conference was to look at harmonizing current approaches to drug regulation and minimizing future divergence of new registration requirements (*Scrip Review,* 1991).

Patent law and protection of intellectual property rights. Patents are the most important of the statutorily created forms of intellectual property for the pharmaceutical industry. According to one source, losses from patent, copyright, and trademark infringement were estimated to cost the industry $6 billion in 1986, resulting in a decrease of $720 to 900 million in R&D spending (Merck and Co., 1988).

Types of protection vary widely between nations. The average time taken to grant a patent also varies by country. The average time it takes for the Japanese Patent Office to grant a patent is about five years from date of filing compared to about twenty months in the United States (*The Japan Times,* 1990). Firms in industrialized countries that have stringent patent protection laws will have more incentive to invest in research and thus will be more productive in discovering NCEs and other new pharmaceutical products.

According to the Pharmaceutical Manufacturer's Association (PMA), "hostile governments, lack of patent protection and well-entrenched patent pirates are reducing the market share and presence of U.S. pharmaceutical companies" in countries such as Bolivia, Colombia, Ecuador, and Peru (PMA, 1990, p. 22). Developing countries in general offer poor patent protection, thus discouraging the diffusion of new drugs into the country.

Pricing and cost-containment policies. Pricing is considered to be one of the "main determinants of margins, research capacities, and internationalization" (*European Chemical News,* 1989, p. 20). Pricing policies of different countries vary depending on national objectives and affect the market attractiveness of a nation, and hence the rate and extent of pharmaceutical innovation and diffusion.

The United States, for example, has to date not implemented price controls on pharmaceuticals and is considered by many to be the country with the "last of the free pricing" (USITC, 1991, pp. 3-19). Pricing controls on pharmaceutical products marketed in the European Community are implemented by almost all of the member states.

According to Redwood (1991), the national pharmaceutical industries of countries with low prices have gradually become less competitive internationally, both as originators of genuinely innovative drugs and in their penetration of international markets.

Redwood (1991) also found a relationship between pricing freedom and trade balance. Of the countries with pricing freedom, only the Netherlands had a trade deficit, whereas no country with product-by-product price control had a pharmaceutical trade surplus. The effect of price control was expressed by Redwood in medical language as follows:

> Drug price control is contra-indicated for high-risk and innovative R&D. Adverse reactions include a propensity to concentrate on the domestic market and to abstain from multinational investment. The result is competitive anemia, one symptom of which is a negative trade balance. (p. 25)

Figure 2.4 illustrates the differential effects of the types of pricing systems (free versus controlled) on pharmaceutical R&D and the political agencies. According to the figure, the interaction of pricing and R&D is not an instant relationship, but one that works its way through the system over the years as a kind of slow motion

FIGURE 2.4. Pricing Systems and Effects on R&D

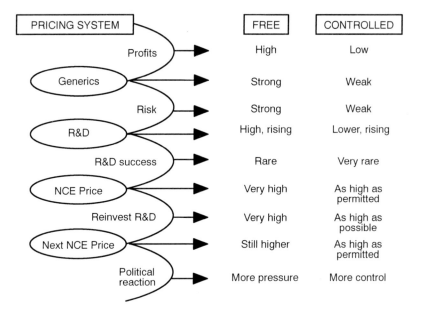

PRICING SYSTEM	FREE	CONTROLLED
Profits	High	Low
Generics	Strong	Weak
Risk	Strong	Weak
R&D	High, rising	Lower, rising
R&D success	Rare	Very rare
NCE Price	Very high	As high as permitted
Reinvest R&D	Very high	As high as possible
Next NCE Price	Still higher	As high as permitted
Political reaction	More pressure	More control

Source: Redwood (1991).

spiral, the twists of which management and the authorities can be responsible for at different times.

Cost containment programs have been implemented by a number of countries such as EC member states, and Japan for health care expenditures. Among other things, these programs are intended to lower the portion of health care expenditures accounted for by pharmaceuticals. The implementation of such programs is becoming more prevalent worldwide as national health care expenditures continue to increase in many countries. Levels of R&D spending in the pharmaceutical industry have been found to decline as a result of price controls and/or cost containment programs on a national level. A reduced level of R&D spending also leads to reduced innovation.

Most developing countries place price controls on pharmaceuticals, reducing perceived market potential and thus diffusion of new products into their markets. This results from the fact that medicines are a "basic need." Drugs account for as much as half of all health care expenditures in these countries (compared with 8 to 10 percent in industrialized countries). Any increase in prices is extremely costly in terms of the health benefits forgone. Policymakers therefore apply tight price controls, sometimes imposing price freezes for extended periods of time (Ballance, Pogany, and Forstner, 1992). Such measures can reduce market attractiveness and thus the supply and demand for pharmaceutical innovations.

Product liability. Product liability law deals with the right of a consumer to sue the manufacturer of a product for injuries caused by a perceived defect in the product. Some countries permit a manufacturer to defend against a product liability suit on the ground that a governmental authority such as the FDA has tested and approved the product as safe. U.S. courts generally do not recognize such a defense and producers face potentially enormous liability even after the government has declared the product to be essentially free of defects (USITC, 1991).

Innovation in the U.S. industry is stunted by concern over potential liability because juries are more likely to find a new product defective than an old, familiar one (Huber, 1988). According to some sources, the specter of product liability exposure has led pharmaceutical companies to shy away from research, particularly in areas such as obstetrics and birth control (Council on Competitiveness, 1991; Swazey, 1991; Lasagna, 1991).

Also, U.S. pharmaceutical companies are finding it more attractive to make their products outside the United States to escape U.S. liability law, thus affecting the supply of new therapies in the United States. Similarly, the diffusion of drugs into the United States from other countries is adversely affected due to stringent product liability measures.

R&D incentives. All the major pharmaceutical producer countries provide at least some government support for pharmaceutical R&D through funding of basic medical research. Federal government support for medical research in the United States continues to exceed funds allocated by other national governments. Developing countries can hardly afford such largesse.

Market/Industry Structure and Competitiveness

Market and/or industry structure can affect both supply and demand of innovative pharmaceuticals. Factors such as level of competition in national as well as international markets, level of diversification in the industry, industry growth, and so on, can have an effect on the supply and diffusion of new drugs.

When the pharmaceutical industry is pictured in global terms, a handful of multinationals are found to dominate. A high degree of concentration prevails in international markets. The top twenty-five companies in the world account for 44 percent of the world market. Fourteen of these companies are based in the United States (Ballance, Pogany, and Forstner, 1992).

Most multinationals are also engaged in a range of activities other than pharmaceuticals. In fact most of the world's largest drug companies obtain the bulk of their revenue from the sale of non-pharmaceutical products. For example, Hoechst, Ciba-Geigy, Bayer, and Rhone-Poulenc are primarily chemical firms with large pharmaceutical departments. Diversification of this type is sometimes regarded as a strategic advantage. That may be true in the sense that the very size of the company offers a degree of financial support which specialized competitors do not enjoy. However, the fact that Merck, Glaxo, and a number of other multinationals depend on pharmaceuticals for more than two-thirds of their total revenue suggests that this advantage, if it exists, is far from decisive (*Financial World*, 1989).

The world's leading pharmaceutical companies are a select group. Entry into this club is very difficult, requiring large teams of researchers as well as a marketing network capable of distributing products on an international or even a global scale.

Product competition in individual markets is not always vigorous. This is because some markets are dominated by a few, relatively efficient drugs that are patent protected. In other instances the patents of the leading brands have expired but the products continue to be leaders due to brand loyalty. Large pharmaceutical firms spend huge sums on product promotion of brand-name drugs, which is clearly a mechanism by which returns on innovation are realized. Some analysts suggest that brand-name loyalty may be a more effective method of guaranteeing high returns than the patent system itself (Lall, 1985).

Demand can also be affected by factors such as the pharmaceutical distribution systems in the country. For example, Japan has a complex wholesale pharmaceutical distribution system and is considered a barrier by several foreign firms. An additional factor that affects market demand (market potential) in Japan is that Japanese physicians both prescribe and dispense medications, gaining income from the difference between their dispensing price and the official reimbursement price. To reach these 180,000 physicians, foreign pharmaceutical firms must supplement their own sales forces with wholesalers' detail men. However, this system indirectly increases the market for pharmaceuticals for firms in Japan, since it provides an incentive to physicians in Japan to prescribe more medications (USITC, 1991).

The degree of market power and the extent of competition do not seem to differ significantly between the industrialized and developing countries. A few companies are world leaders and occupy prominent positions in the markets of both country groups. Nevertheless, the implications for policymakers and consumers in developing countries are worrying. The domestic industry in these countries is relatively weak and consists exclusively of small firms that can pose no challenge to the multinationals. This can mean that markets are relatively vulnerable to the possible abuse of market power (Redwood, 1988).

Innovation-Specific Factors and Competitiveness

The market potential of the therapeutic category to which the new chemical entity belongs will affect the level of R&D investment and consequently the number of new chemical entities introduced in a given time period. For example, the leading therapeutic category in terms of R&D investment in 1989 was anti-infectives, with 1,215 products in development worldwide. Neurologicals, anticancer, and cardiovasculars were the other leading therapeutic categories. These were also the categories that topped the list in terms of worldwide revenue (*Scrip*, 1990).

Therapeutic category of innovation would also determine the nature of demand for the new chemical entity. Disease patterns may vary widely between temperate and tropical nations. Some drugs will have general clinical relevance across all nations. Others will have a limited market because they treat medical conditions that are relatively rare and specific to particular countries. The drugs that have a universal relevance are likely to be introduced into many nations.

For example, in 1989, cardiovascular and central nervous system (CNS) products were the two leading categories of ethical drugs in terms of U.S. sales, whereas anti-infective and cardiovascular products were the two leading categories overseas (USITC, 1991). Table 2.3 lists the environmental conditions and factors that affect global competitiveness in the pharmaceutical industry.

TABLE 2.3. Environmental Conditions and Global Pharmaceutical Competitiveness

Environment	Factors
(1) Demographic Environment	Population density, life expectancy, birth rate, composition/distribution of population, etc.
(2) Social Environment	Health care systems, nature of consumer demand, dispensing practices of physicians, etc.
(3) Economic Environment	GNP/capita, per capita income, expenditure patterns on health care, etc.
(4) Political Environment	Government involvement in business, developmental priorities, ideological orientation, etc.
(5) Legal Environment	Regulatory approval times, patent laws, pricing policies, product liability, R&D tax laws, etc.
(6) Market/Industry Environment	Market concentration, industry focus, industry growth, market size, distribution systems, etc.
(7) Innovation-Specific Factors	Demand for therapeutic category.

Developing Country Competitiveness Issues

As discussed above, international competitiveness in the pharmaceutical industry depends on a complex interaction of demographic, economic, social, cultural, market, and legal characteristics. The many hurdles, delays, and problems encountered by the Japanese in countering competition from the traditionally dominating multinationals in the United States and Western Europe are instructive when attention turns to developing countries.

If Japan, a country with a huge domestic market, ample financial resources, and abundant technical skills, requires such a long time to build up a competitive pharmaceutical industry, what are the strategic options available to firms in developing countries?

The choices are comparatively few, primarily because producers in developing countries lack research expertise. China seems to be one exception. The country's growing links with firms in industrialized countries reflect the latter's interest in developing retail and OTC products from traditional Chinese herbal remedies. Some foreign participants hope to make use of Chinese research on biological agents which they would convert into drugs.

Few firms in developing countries have such a research option. Only a handful have actually discovered an NCE and the instances of collaboration between pairs of firms that are owned and operated in developing countries are few. A multinational usually initiates such contacts; the objective is invariably to gain market access. The multinationals' early moves into developing countries allowed little or no role for local industry. The growth of domestic demand and the lure of larger public-health budgets has made the markets of at least a few developing countries more attractive investment sites. That is the case in several Asian countries where demand for medicines is growing by more than 10 percent each year (Ballance, Pogany, and Forstner, 1992).

Many developing countries such as India recognize patents only for processes. Some of the companies in India specialize in developing new chemical processes, yielding drugs that are identical to those produced (at much greater expense) by multinationals. The Indian firms begin by selling their new products domestically; later they scale up operations to cut manufacturing costs.

The foreign markets which they select as targets are countries that recognize process patents but not patents on the product itself. By the time the companies are ready to export they can often sell the drugs at less than a tenth the price charged by competitors in industrialized countries. This is one of the few means by which developing countries can compete against multinationals. However, the growth of generic markets and the many drugs that will soon come off patent mean that a greater portion of the world's markets could soon be open to producers in developing countries.

The Southeast Asian market is also increasing in its importance both as a competitor—with respect to new multinationals from Southeast Asia—and as a potential investment area for American, Japanese, and European firms. According to Howe (1992), "to be globally competitive into the twenty-first century, pharmaceutical companies will have to be successful in the Southeast Asian market" (p. 8).

The Southeast Asian region represents the fourth largest market for pharmaceuticals and the fastest growing market in the world (Howe, 1992). The market tripled in size between 1989 and 1991 and expanded as a base for production as well as sales. The region, together with China, currently consumes approximately 8 percent of the world's pharmaceuticals and accounts for over 5 percent of U.S. pharmaceutical exports (see Table 2.4).

TABLE 2.4. Asian Pharmaceutical Markets by Size

Market	Size (in U.S. $ millions, rounded)
Total world	120,000
Japan	33,000 (27.5% of world)
Southeast Asia	
China	4,200
South Korea	2,448
Taiwan	852
Philippines	589
Indonesia	536
Thailand	478
Hong Kong	154
Malaysia	146
Singapore	73
Total Southeast Asia	9,476 (7.9% of world)

Source: The IMS Drug Market Manual (Asia), 1990.

Among the Southeast Asian countries likely to emerge as powerful competitors in the future are South Korea, Indonesia, Singapore, Taiwan, and China. Singapore, South Korea, and Taiwan, for example, have explicitly named biotechnology as a high priority. To foster development, these countries have created technology centers, offered tax incentives, and tried to improve basic research in order to develop more competent scientists.

GLOBAL STRATEGIC PERSPECTIVES

Strategic management of the global supply and demand factors that affect pharmaceutical sales is crucially important for multinational managers for sustained international competitive advantage. Some of the strategies that were identified in the literature and are applicable to the pharmaceutical industry will now be discussed.

Core Competencies

According to Prahalad and Hamel (1990), the most powerful way to prevail in global competition in the 1990s will depend on the ability to exploit core competencies. Core competencies are "the collective learning in the organization, especially the coordination of diverse production skills and integration of multiple streams of technology" (p. 82).

Three important characteristics of a core competency in a corporation are: (1) it provides potential access to a wide variety of markets, (2) it should make a significant contribution to the perceived customer benefits of the end product, and (3) it should be difficult for competitors to imitate. Also, core competencies are built through a process of continuous improvement and enhancement that may span a decade or longer.

Bogner and Thomas (1992) studied the core competencies in the pharmaceutical industry using a sample of nine firms for intensive case study. They identified two types of competencies in the pharmaceutical industry: (1) competencies in R&D, and (2) competencies in marketing and promotion which include the ability to handle regulatory requirements. Further, they found that the environment in these areas is constantly changing and that not all firms pick up on these changes. Additionally, firm-specific learning with respect to technology and marketing is critical for long-term maintenance of competitive advantage.

With respect to core competencies in R&D in the pharmaceutical industry, the technological areas that successful firms exploited for discovering new drugs, from the 1870s to the present have been in organic chemistry, fermentation and soil screening (1940s), rational drug design (1970s), and biotechnology (1980s). Competencies in marketing and promotion have changed from direct selling to physicians (1950s), to blockbuster marketing (1980s), to specialized selling and handling of regulatory requirements.

Comparative Advantage-Based Competitive Advantage

A second concept made popular in international strategic management by Kogut (1985) and one which particularly applies to this research study, is the concept of comparative advantage-based competitive advantage. It implies the design of international strategies based on the interplay between the comparative advantages of countries and the competitive advantages of firms.

Comparative advantage, sometimes referred to as location-specific advantage, influences the decision of where to source and market. Competitive advantage, sometimes referred to as firm-specific advantage, influences the decision of what activities and technologies along the value-added chain a firm should concentrate its resources in, that is, the core competency of the firm. For example, a U.S.-based pharmaceutical firm with a core competency in a certain therapeutic area could choose to locate in a country where there is a greater demand for that therapeutic category and where the approval procedure for new drugs is less stringent than that of the U.S. FDA. This would enable the firm to exploit the comparative advantage of the foreign country as well as its own competitive advantage. Several U.S. companies, for example, with core competencies in R&D choose to locate their R&D facilities in the United Kingdom rather than the United States because of the faster approval process in the United Kingdom.

Differences in comparative advantages of countries with respect to pharmaceuticals arise due to differences in institutional, cultural, economic, legal, political, market, and industry environments. These differences result in differing factor costs, thus contributing to the competitive advantage of firms that are able to take advantage of the lower factor costs.

Differences in the firm-specific advantages or core competencies arise depending on which activities along the value-added chain the firm has invested in learning. The value-added chain for pharmaceuticals is illustrated in Figure 2.5. By examining the value-added chain it can be determined which activities will be placed in countries where the comparative advantage is most favorable, thus exploiting differences in input markets.

According to Ghoshal (1987), the same can be applied to exploiting differences in output markets, that is, different countries offer

FIGURE 2.5. Value-Added Chain for Pharmaceuticals

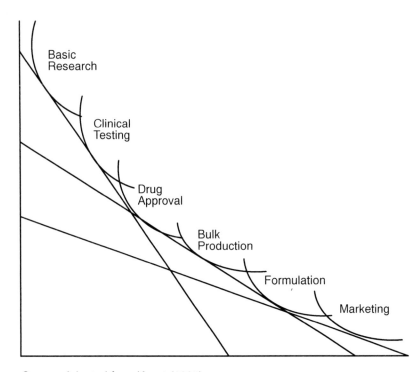

Source: Adapted from Kogut (1985).

different comparative advantages in terms of differences in consumer tastes and preferences, distribution systems, government regulations, and so on. It is also important to remember that comparative advantage is a dynamic concept and can change with changes in government policies and economic or social conditions.

Collaborate to Compete

In recent years, several experts have studied the effectiveness of alliances in international business and found them to be an important weapon of competitive advantage in the global competitive arena (Hamel, Doz, and Prahalad, 1989; Harrigan, 1987; Ohmae, 1989). According to Hamel, Doz, and Prahalad, "it takes so much money to develop new products and to penetrate new markets that few companies can go it alone in every situation" (p. 133).

The accelerating rate of technological change and the broader range of technological capabilities that firms must possess are also reasons for alliances between firms. Domestic and international mergers, joint ventures, and strategic alliances proliferated in the global pharmaceutical industry in the 1980s. According to one source, approximately 131 pharmaceutical firms announced acquisitions or strategic alliances in the first six months of 1990, compared with a total of fifty-one in 1989 and fifty-six in 1988 (*Medical Advertising Newsletter,* 1990).

The reasons are increasing R&D costs, pressure by governments to contain health costs, and longer drug approval procedures in many countries. One example of an early strategic alliance was the 1983 copromotion agreement between Glaxo and Hoffman-LaRoche. Under the agreement, Hoffman-LaRoche marketed Glaxo's antiulcer product Zantac in the United States, under the Glaxo trade name, for a percentage of the sales revenue generated. The result was beneficial to both companies, with Glaxo establishing name recognition in the United States and Hoffman-LaRoche generating extra revenue to compensate for the 1985 expiration of its patent on Valium.

France, dominated by domestic companies and involvement of the government in pricing approval, has led many overseas companies to forge alliances with French companies. Italy's market is slightly less nationalistic, but the need to develop a close relationship with governmental agencies to obtain more timely approval and attractive pricing makes marketing alliances with domestic companies attractive.

According to Shan and Hamilton (1991), such international cooperative ventures provide a firm with access to country-specific advantages embedded in its partners. Therefore "from this perspective, international cooperative relationships may be viewed as a vehicle to tap into the comparative advantages of countries" (p. 419).

In their study of a sample of domestic and international cooperative relationships of Japanese firms in the biotechnology industry, Shan and Hamilton found country-specific advantage to be a significant variable in explaining differences between cooperative relationships with partners of different countries. They concluded that interfirm cooperation has implications for international competitiveness of both firms and nations in high-technology industries.

Chapter 3

Methodology

This chapter has five sections. The first section presents an overview of the research design and the conceptual model used in the study. The second section presents the research questions, the executive survey, and the responses. The third section discusses the path models that were tested in the study and the constructs, measures, and data sources used. The fourth section consists of the hypotheses proposed for both models. The final section is a discussion of the statistical technique used (EQS) to analyze the models.

OVERVIEW OF RESEARCH DESIGN AND CONCEPTUAL MODEL

For the purpose of developing the conceptual framework, the research design, and the hypotheses, three streams of literature were reviewed. These were: (1) theoretical and conceptual perspectives on national competitiveness, (2) competitiveness in the global pharmaceutical industry, and (3) global strategic management perspectives.

The conceptual model used to develop the statistical path models in the study is shown in Figure 2.1. The model illustrates a number of supply and demand related factors that affect global competitiveness in the pharmaceutical industry. The demand for ethical pharmaceuticals is determined by demographic and socioeconomic factors. Government policies and programs also affect the demand for drugs, directly or indirectly. An important factor affecting the supply of ethical pharmaceuticals is R&D activity, that is, the level and productivity of R&D spending. Government actions ranging from macroeconomic policies to treatment of product liability and regulatory controls exert direct and indirect effects (positive and negative) on the ability of firms and the industry as a whole to produce pharmaceuticals.

Besides a review of the literature, talks with industry experts and responses from an executive survey conducted before the actual data collection provided insights into development of the constructs and measures for the study. Data was obtained from secondary sources, mainly from the *Scrip League Tables* and governmental publications such as the United Nations' *World Development Reports*. Pharmaceutical industry data for a total of twenty-seven countries were used in this study. Of these, fifteen are industrialized countries and twelve are developing countries. Two-group analysis was done to examine differences in competitiveness factors between the industrialized (I) and developing (D) nation pharmaceutical industries.

RESEARCH QUESTIONS

The broad objective of the study, as indicated in its title, was to examine the factors affecting global competitiveness in the pharmaceutical industry. The literature review, expert opinions, and the executive survey responses revealed that two important factors underly global competitiveness in the pharmaceutical industry. These are: (1) ability to innovate and (2) ability to market innovations worldwide. These observations led to the following three research objectives or questions:

1. Which country factors stimulate or inhibit a nation's pharmaceutical industry to be globally innovative?
2. Which country factors stimulate or inhibit diffusion of pharmaceutical innovations into its markets?
3. Are there differences between industrialized and developing countries with respect to factors that affect innovation and global competitiveness in the pharmaceutical industry?

Executive Survey

As mentioned above, a survey of executives working for multinational pharmaceutical companies was carried out to determine the factors that affect global competitiveness in the pharmaceutical industry.

A sample of about forty-five multinational pharmaceutical companies was chosen from the 1992 *Pharmaceutical Marketers Directory*.

Two executives from each company were selected to answer the survey. One of the executives was the CEO or president of the company and the second executive selected was the director for market research. Therefore a total of ninety surveys were mailed out.

The survey was one page long and consisted of two open-ended questions (see Figure 3.1). There was also a cover letter explaining the nature of the study, with an assurance that all replies would be kept confidential. The respondents were also promised a report of the study results if interested. The executives had the option of filling out the one-page questionnaire and simply faxing the sheet back to the number provided or mailing it back in an envelope to the address provided. The questionnaire also indicated that handwritten responses were acceptable. The above measures were designed to increase the response rate by making the task as simple as possible for the executives.

Survey Responses

The executive responses obtained served to confirm the observations from the literature regarding factors affecting global competitiveness in the pharmaceutical industry. Some of the responses from the survey are presented below.

1. In your opinion, what factors make a country's pharmaceutical industry globally competitive?

   * Innovation—far and away the single most important factor.
   * Resources to competitively access various markets.
   * Innovative differentiated products.
   * The quality and scope of medical research.
   * Ability to distribute products on a global scale.

2. In your opinion, which are the important criteria that a firm must consider when selecting foreign markets for introducing their products?

   * market potential
   * regulatory environment
   * competition
   * reimbursement/pricing systems
   * patent protection
   * return on investment, etc.

FIGURE 3.1. Executive Survey

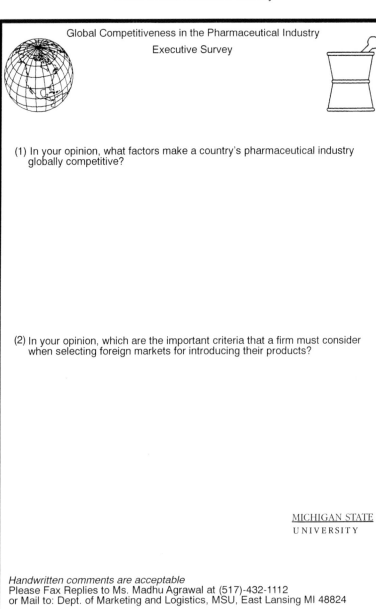

Global Competitiveness in the Pharmaceutical Industry

Executive Survey

(1) In your opinion, what factors make a country's pharmaceutical industry globally competitive?

(2) In your opinion, which are the important criteria that a firm must consider when selecting foreign markets for introducing their products?

MICHIGAN STATE
UNIVERSITY

Handwritten comments are acceptable
Please Fax Replies to Ms. Madhu Agrawal at (517)-432-1112
or Mail to: Dept. of Marketing and Logistics, MSU, East Lansing MI 48824

MODEL DEVELOPMENT

Path models were developed to test the research questions. Based on the conceptual model, two models were designed to test the supply (innovation) and the demand (diffusion) factors affecting global competitiveness in the pharmaceutical industry.

The Global Innovation Model (GIM)

Figure 3.2a illustrates the global innovation model. As shown, three major factors are proposed as affecting the extent of investment in innovation by a country's pharmaceutical industry. These factors are: (a) the economic environment, (b) the regulatory environment, and (c) the market/industry structure. The market/industry environment is also directly affected by the country's economic environment.

The extent of innovation investment is proposed as affecting both outbound foreign investment by a country's pharmaceutical industry and its success in global innovation. Global innovation is also hypothesized as being affected directly by the extent of foreign investment. Global innovation in turn is proposed as directly affecting the global competitiveness of the country's pharmaceutical industry.

FIGURE 3.2a. The Global Innovation Model

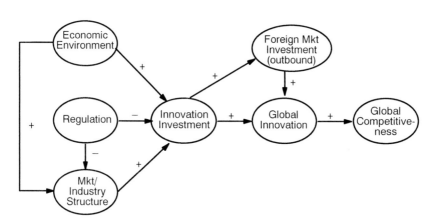

The Global Diffusion Model (GDM)

Figure 3.2b illustrates the global diffusion model. As shown, three major factors are proposed as affecting the market potential for pharmaceutical innovations in a country. These factors are: (a) the economic environment, (b) the regulatory environment, and (c) the market/industry structure.

The market potential is proposed as affecting *inbound* foreign investment in the country's pharmaceutical industry as well as global diffusion of innovations into the country. Global diffusion is also hypothesized as being affected directly by the extent of inbound pharmaceutical foreign investment. An additional factor hypothesized as affecting global diffusion is global innovation. That is, extent of NCE diffusion into a country is directly affected by the extent of innovation by the country.

The individual constructs, measures, and data sources for both the above models are discussed below.

Constructs, Measures, and Data Sources

The Global Innovation Model

Economic environment. As discussed in Chapter 2, countries on a higher level of economic development are characterized by more

FIGURE 3.2b. The Global Diffusion Model

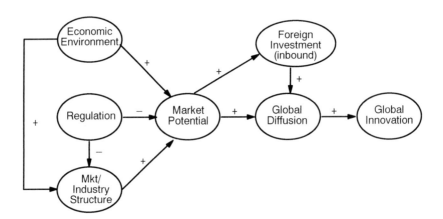

innovative pharmaceutical industries compared to countries that are economically less developed. Several indicators are available by which the economic status of a country can be assessed. Two indicators or measures used in this study were:

1. GNP per capita (GNP): The average gross national product per country's population measured in U.S. dollars for the years under study.
2. Population (POP): The average absolute population for the country for the years under study.

Regulatory environment. This is one of the most important factors affecting global innovation. Chapter 2 reviews the literature and empirical studies demonstrating the effects of various regulatory mechanisms on innovation in the pharmaceutical industry. This study uses two regulatory measures:

1. Price regulation (PRICEREG): This is the extent of price control on pharmaceuticals exerted by the government of the country. A seven-point scale, where 1 reflects low price control and 7 reflects high price control, is used to measure price control.
2. Approval time (APPTIME): This is the time taken by the drug regulatory agencies to approve an application of a new pharmaceutical product or NCE for marketing in the country. This is measured using a seven-point scale, where 1 reflects short approval time and 7 reflects long approval time.

The above measures for regulatory environment are subjective measures determined by the researcher. Although objective values for PRICEREG and APPTIME would have been desirable, the unavailability coupled with the unreliability (due to differences in reporting systems of countries) of the existing objective data on the above indicators made it necessary to resort to subjective measures. An abundance of anecdotal and other information was available to facilitate development of the subjective measures for PRICEREG and APPTIME.

Market and industry structure. As was discussed in Chapter 2, the structural aspects of the market and industry can significantly affect the country's innovation potential in pharmaceuticals. Four indicators of market and industry structure were used in this study:

1. Market size (MKTSIZE): This was measured as the average annual sales (in U.S. dollars) of pharmaceuticals for the country for the years under study.
2. Industry focus (INDFOCUS): This was measured as the average percentage ratio of pharmaceutical sales to total sales for the country's industry.
3. Industry growth (INDGRWTH): This was measured as the average annual percentage change in pharmaceutical sales for the country's industry.
4. Industry concentration (INDCONC): This was measured as the percentage of total pharmaceutical sales accounted by the top twenty-five firms in the industry for the country.

Innovation investment. This is the investment in R&D activities by a country's industry. It is a significant predictor of innovative success, since the greater the investment in innovation, the greater should be the success with respect to discovery of new products. One indicator was used for the above construct:

1. R&D expenditure (R&DEXPD): This was the average annual expenditure (in U.S. dollars) on pharmaceutical research and development by the country's industry.

Outbound foreign investment. Internationalization by a country's pharmaceutical industry is a significant indicator of its size and research potential and has been shown to be positively linked to innovation in most high-technology industries. Two indicators were used to measure outbound foreign investment:

1. Absolute foreign investment (FRGINVST): This was the average annual foreign sales (in U.S. dollars) of pharmaceuticals by the country's industry.
2. Foreign commitment (FRGCOMM): This was the average percentage ratio of foreign pharmaceutical sales to total pharmaceutical (foreign + domestic) sales for the country's pharmaceutical industry.

Global innovation. This construct reflects the success of the country's industry in developing successfully a new pharmaceutical or NCE. This was measured as:

1. Number of NCEs developed (INNOVAT): This was measured as the total number of NCEs developed by a country's industry for the years under study.

Global competitiveness. This reflects the market power of the country's industry in the global market. This was measured as:

1. Global Sales (GBLSALES): This was measured as the average annual worldwide pharmaceutical sales (in U.S. dollars) by the country's pharmaceutical industry.

Table 3.1a lists the constructs, measures, and data sources used in the global innovation model.

The Global Diffusion Model

Four constructs used in the GIM are also used in the diffusion model (see Figures 3.2a and 3.2b). The same indicators were also used. Therefore only those constructs and corresponding measures that are different are discussed below:

Market potential. As discussed in Chapter 2, market potential or market attractiveness is a significant determinant of the country's ability to attract companies desirous of introducing NCEs in that country. This was measured as follows:

1. Market potential (MKTPOT): This was measured as the average annual sales (in U.S. dollars) of pharmaceuticals for the country for the years under study.

Inbound foreign investment. The extent of pharmaceutical foreign investment in a country will positively affect the number of new pharmaceuticals introduced into the country every year. This construct was measured as:

1. INFRGN: The average annual value of pharmaceutical imports (in U.S. dollars) into the country.

TABLE 3.1a. Constructs, Measures, and Data Sources: The Global Innovation Model

Constructs	Measures	Sources
1. Macroeconomic Environment	1. GNP per capita (GNP)	*World Development Reports*, UN Publication.
	2. Population (POP)	*World Development Reports*, UN Publication.
2. Regulation	1. Price control (PRICEREG)	Author's estimates, various sources.
	2. Approval time (APPTIME)	Author's estimates, various sources.
3. Market/Industry Structure	1. Market size (MKTSIZE)	*Scrip Review* (various issues).
	2. Industry focus (INDFOCUS)	*Scrip League Tables*.
	3. Industry growth (INDGRWTH)	*Scrip League Tables*.
	4. Industry concentration (IND-CONC)	Ballance, Pogany, and Forstner (1992).
4. Innovation Investment	1. R&D Expenditure (R&DEXPD)	*Scrip League Tables*.
5. Foreign Market Investment (Outbound)	1. Absolute foreign investment (FRGINVST)	*Scrip League Tables*.
	2. Foreign commitment (FRGCOMM)	*Scrip League Tables*.
6. Global Innovation	1. Number of NCEs developed (INNOVAT)	*Scrip Review* (various issues).
7. Global Competitive-ness	1. Global Sales (GBLSALES)	*Scrip League Tables*.

TABLE 3.1b. Constructs, Measures, and Data Sources: The Global Diffusion Model

Constructs	Measures	Sources
1. Macroeconomic Environment	1. GNP per capita (GNP)	*World Development Reports*, UN Publication.
	2. Population (POP)	*World Development Reports*, UN Publication.
2. Regulation	1. Price control (PRICEREG)	Author's estimates, various sources.
	2. Approval time (APPTIME)	Author's estimates, various sources.
3. Market/Industry Structure	1. Industry focus (INDFOCUS)	*Scrip League Tables*.
	2. Industry growth (INDGRWTH)	*Scrip League Tables*.
	3. Industry concentration (IND-CONC)	Ballance, Pogany, and Forstner (1992).
4. Market Potential	1. market potential (MKTPOT)	*Scrip Review* (various issues).
5. Foreign Market In-vestment (Inbound)	1. Foreign imports (INFRGN)	*World Trade Annual*.
6. Global Diffusion	1. # of NCEs introduced (DIFF)	*Scrip Review* (various issues).
7. Global Innovation	1. # of NCEs developed (INNOVAT)	*Scrip Review* (various issues).

Global diffusion. This construct indicates the recipient country's attractiveness as a market for introduction of new pharmaceutical products. This was measured as:

1. DIFF: The total number of NCEs introduced into the country for the years under study.

Table 3.1b lists the constructs, measures, and data sources used in the global diffusion model.

Data Sources, Sample Size, and Time Frame

All data used in this study were obtained from secondary sources because most data were objective. These sources were identified after a thorough review of the literature—both academic and trade journals; consultation with industry experts such as the Pharmaceutical Manufacturers Association; and talks with pharmaceutical market research firms such as Scrip, IMS, and so on. Tables 3.1a and 3.1b list the data sources used for the measures in each of the models.

The total sample size used in the study was twenty-seven countries (see Table 3.2). Data from 202 multinationals representing these countries was aggregated to obtain country-level estimates. The time frame over which the data were examined was a four-year period (1990 to 1994). This time frame was considered appropriate, as a

TABLE 3.2. Countries in Sample

Argentina	Japan
Australia	Korea
Belgium	Netherlands
Canada	New Zealand
China	Norway
Denmark	Portugal
Finland	South Africa
France	Spain
Germany	Sweden
Hungary	Switzerland
India	Turkey
Indonesia	United Kingdom
Israel	United States
Italy	

longer time frame would involve confounding effects due to the dynamic environmental changes taking place in the industry before 1990. A shorter time frame would have been ineffective in measuring effects such as innovation and diffusion, which take place over a period of several months.

HYPOTHESES

A total of thirty hypotheses corresponding to thirty different path relationships were proposed for the global innovation model. Since several of the constructs in the global diffusion model were the same as in the innovation model, resulting in similar paths, only seven unique hypotheses (paths) were applicable to the global diffusion model.

The hypotheses were developed from a review of the literature and results of previous empirical studies. Tables 3.3a and 3.3b list the hypothesized paths, their expected significance, and direction for the global innovation model and the global diffusion model respectively. The rationale for each of the hypotheses and the actual result is discussed in detail in Chapter 4.

In order to test the above hypotheses, a total of thirty-two program runs were carried out for the global innovation model and twelve program runs for the global diffusion model. The number of program runs reflects the number of measures used and the paths tested. Tables 3.4a and 3.4b list the combination of variables used in each run for the global innovation and the global diffusion models respectively.

STATISTICAL METHOD OF ANALYSIS—EQS

EQS is a structural equation modeling (SEM) software that was used for statistical analysis. Structural equation modeling is an extension of several multivariate techniques (such as multiple regression and factor analysis). It provides a straightforward method of dealing with multiple dependence relationships simultaneously while providing statistical efficiency (Hayduk, 1987).

TABLE 3.3a. Hypotheses: The Global Innovation Model

Paths			Expected Direction	Expected Significance
H1:	GNP	——> MKTSIZE	+	significant
H2:	GNP	——> R&DEXPD	+	significant
H3:	PRICEREG	——> MKTSIZE	−	significant
H4:	PRICEREG	——> R&DEXPD	−	significant
H5:	MKTSIZE	——> R&DEXPD	+	significant
H6:	R&DEXPD	——> FRGINVST	+	significant
H7:	R&DEXPD	——> INNOVAT	+	significant
H8:	FRGINVST	——> INNOVAT	+	significant
H9:	INNOVAT	——> GBLSALES	+	significant
H10:	GNP	——> INDFOCUS	+	insignificant
H11:	PRICEREG	——> INDFOCUS	−	significant
H12:	INDFOCUS	——> R&DEXPD	+	significant
H13:	GNP	——> INDGRWTH	+	insignificant
H14:	PRICEREG	——> INDGRWTH	−	significant
H15:	INDGRWTH	——> R&DEXPD	+	insignificant
H16:	GNP	——> INDCONC	−	insignificant
H17:	PRICEREG	——> INDCONC	+	insignificant
H18:	INDCONC	——> R&DEXPD	+	insignificant
H19:	POP	——> MKTSIZE	+	significant
H20:	POP	——> R&DEXPD	+	significant
H21:	APPTIME	——> MKTSIZE	−	significant
H22:	APPTIME	——> R&DEXPD	−	significant
H23:	OP	——> INDFOCUS	+	significant
H24:	APPTIME	——> INDFOCUS	−	insignificant
H25:	POP	——> INDGRWTH	+	insignificant
H26:	APPTIME	——> INDGRWTH	−	significant
H27:	POP	——> INDCONC	−	insignificant
H28:	APPTIME	——> INDCONC	+	insignificant
H29:	R&DEXPD	——> FRGCOMM	+	significant
H30:	FRGCOMM	——> INNOVAT	−	insignificant

TABLE 3.3b. Hypotheses: The Global Diffusion Model

Paths			Expected Direction	Expected Significance
H1:	INDFOCUS	——> MKTPOT	+	significant
H2:	INDGRWTH	——> MKTPOT	+	significant
H3:	INDCONC	——> MKTPOT	−	significant
H4:	MKTPOT	——> INFRGN	+	significant
H5:	MKTPOT	——> DIFF	+	significant
H6:	INFRGN	——> DIFF	+	significant
H7:	INNOVAT	——> DIFF	+	significant

TABLE 3.4a. Program Runs for the Global Innovation Model

(1)	v1=gnp;	v2=pricereg;	vv3=mktsize;	v4=r&dexpd;	v5=frginvst;	v6=innovat;	v7=gblsales
(2)	v1=gnp;	v2=pricereg;	v3=mktfocus;	v4=r&dexpd;	v5=frginvst;	v6=innovat;	v7=gblsales
(3)	v1=gnp;	v2=pricereg;	v3=mktgrwth;	v4=r&dexpd;	v5=frginvst;	v6=innovat;	v7=gblsales
(4)	v1=gnp;	v2=pricereg;	v3=mktconc;	v4=r&dexpd;	v5=frginvst;	v6=innovat;	v7=gblsales
(5)	v1=gnp;	v2=apptime;	v3=mktsize;	v4=r&dexpd;	v5=frginvst;	v6=innovat;	v7=gblsales
(6)	v1=gnp;	v2=apptime;	v3=mktfocus;	v4=r&dexpd;	v5=frginvst;	v6=innovat;	v7=gblsales
(7)	v1=gnp;	v2=apptime;	v3=mktgrwth;	v4=r&dexpd;	v5=frginvst;	v6=innovat;	v7=gblsales
(8)	v1=gnp;	v2=apptime;	v3=mktconc;	v4=r&dexpd;	v5=frginvst;	v6=innovat;	v7=gblsales
(9)	v1=pop;	v2=pricereg;	v3=mktsize;	v4=r&dexpd;	v5=frginvst;	v6=innovat;	v7=gblsales
(10)	v1=pop;	v2=pricereg;	v3=mktfocus;	v4=r&dexpd;	v5=frginvst;	v6=innovat;	v7=gblsales
(11)	v1=pop;	v2=pricereg;	v3=mktfocus;	v4=r&dexpd;	v5=frginvst;	v6=innovat;	v7=gblsales
(12)	v1=pop;	v2=pricereg;	v3=mktconc;	v4=r&dexpd;	v5=frginvst;	v6=innovat;	v7=gblsales
(13)	v1=pop;	v2=apptime;	v3=mktsize;	v4=r&dexpd;	v5=frginvst;	v6=innovat;	v7=gblsales
(14)	v1=pop;	v2=apptime;	v3=mktfocus;	v4=r&dexpd;	v5=frginvst;	v6=innovat;	v7=gblsales
(15)	v1=pop;	v2=apptime;	v3=mktgrwth;	v4=r&dexpd;	v5=frginvst;	v6=innovat;	v7=gblsales
(16)	v1=pop;	v2=apptime;	v3=mktconc;	v4=r&dexpd;	v5=frginvst;	v6=innovat;	v7=gblsales
(17)	v1=gnp;	v2=pricereg;	v3=mktsize;	v4=r&dexpd;	v5=frgcomm;	v6=innovat;	v7=gblsales
(18)	v1=gnp;	v2=pricereg;	v3=mktfocus;	v4=r&dexpd;	v5=frgcomm;	v6=innovat;	v7=gblsales
(19)	v1=gnp;	v2=pricereg;	v3=mktgrwth;	v4=r&dexpd;	v5=frgcomm;	v6=innovat;	v7=gblsales
(20)	v1=gnp;	v2=pricereg;	v3=mktconc;	v4=r&dexpd;	v5=frgcomm;	v6=innovat;	v7=gblsales
(21)	v1=gnp;	v2=apptime;	v3=mktsize;	v4=r&dexpd;	v5=frgcomm;	v6=innovat;	v7=gblsales
(22)	v1=gnp;	v2=apptime;	v3=mktfocus;	v4=r&dexpd;	v5=frgcomm;	v6=innovat;	v7=gblsales
(23)	v1=gnp;	v2=apptime;	v3=mktgrwth;	v4=r&dexpd;	v5=frgcomm;	v6=innovat;	v7=gblsales
(24)	v1=gnp;	v2=apptime;	v3=mktconc;	v4=r&dexpd;	v5=frgcomm;	v6=innovat;	v7=gblsales
(25)	v1=pop;	v2=pricereg;	v3=mktsize;	v4=r&dexpd;	v5=frgcomm;	v6=innovat;	v7=gblsales
(26)	v1=pop;	v2=pricereg;	v3=mktfocus;	v4=r&dexpd;	v5=frgcomm;	v6=innovat;	v7=gblsales
(27)	v1=pop;	v2=pricereg;	v3=mktgrwth;	v4=r&dexpd;	v5=frgcomm;	v6=innovat;	v7=gblsales
(28)	v1=pop;	v2=pricereg;	v3=mktconc;	v4=r&dexpd;	v5=frgcomm;	v6=innovat;	v7=gblsales
(29)	v1=pop;	v2=apptime;	v3=mktsize;	v4=r&dexpd;	v5=frgcomm;	v6=innovat;	v7=gblsales
(30)	v1=pop;	v2=apptime;	v3=mktfocus;	v4=r&dexpd;	v5=frgcomm;	v6=innovat;	v7=gblsales
(31)	v1=pop;	v2=apptime;	v3=mktgrwth;	v4=r&dexpd;	v5=frgcomm;	v6=innovat;	v7=gblsales
(32)	v1=pop;	v2=apptime;	v3=mktconc;	v4=r&dexpd;	v5=frgcomm;	v6=innovat;	v7=gblsales

TABLE 3.4b. Program Runs for the Global Diffusion Model

(1)	v1=gnp;	v2=pricereg;	v3=indfocus;	v4=mktpot;	v5=infrgn;	v6=diff;	v7=innovat
(2)	v1=gnp;	v2=pricereg;	v3=indgrwth;	v4=mktpot;	v5=infrgn;	v6=diff;	v7=innovat
(3)	v1=gnp;	v2=pricereg;	v3=indconc;	v4=mktpot;	v5=infrgn;	v6=diff;	v7=innovat
(4)	v1=gnp;	v2=apptime;	v3=indfocus;	v4=mktpot;	v5=infrgn;	v6=diff;	v7=innovat
(5)	v1=gnp;	v2=apptime;	v3=indgrwth;	v4=mktpot;	v5=infrgn;	v6=diff;	v7=innovat
(6)	v1=gnp;	v2=apptime;	v3=indconc;	v4=mktpot;	v5=infrgn;	v6=diff;	v7=innovat
(7)	v1=pop;	v2=pricereg;	v3=indfocus;	v4=mktpot;	v5=infrgn;	v6=diff;	v7=innovat
(8)	v1=pop;	v2=pricereg;	v3=indgrwth;	v4=mktpot;	v5=infrgn;	v6=diff;	v7=innovat
(9)	v1=pop;	v2=pricereg;	v3=indconc;	v4=mktpot;	v5=infrgn;	v6=diff;	v7=innovat
(10)	v1=pop;	v2=apptime;	v3=indfocus;	v4=mktpot;	v5=infrgn;	v6=diff;	v7=innovat
(11)	v1=pop;	v2=apptime;	v3=indgrwth;	v4=mktpot;	v5=infrgn;	v6=diff;	v7=innovat
(12)	v1=pop;	v2=apptime;	v3=indconc;	v4=mktpot;	v5=infrgn;	v6=diff;	v7=innovat

Uses of Structural Equation Modeling

1. Understand the role of causal relationships in statistical analysis.
2. Represent a series of causal relationships in a path diagram.
3. Translate a path diagram into a set of equations for estimation.
4. Assess overall model fit using goodness-of-fit measures.

Steps in Structural Equation Modeling

The following steps are involved in analyzing a path model using structural equation modeling.

Assessing identification of the model. Very often during the estimation process, the computer program is likely to "blow up", that is, produce meaningless or illogical results, producing what are called "identification problems." In simple terms, an identification problem is the inability of the proposed model to generate unique estimates. Usually there are three sources of identification problems that need to be explored and corrected: (1) a large number of estimated coefficients relative to the number of covariances or correlations, indicated by a small number of degrees of freedom; (2) the use of reciprocal effects (two-way causal arrows between two constructs); or (3) failure to fix the scale of a construct.

Evaluating goodness of fit. Structural equation modeling (SEM) shares three assumptions with the other multivariate methods: independent observations, random sampling of respondents, and the linearity of all relationships. In addition, SEM is more sensitive to the distributional characteristics of the data, particularly the departure from multivariate normality or a strong kurtosis (skewness) in the data. A lack of multivariate normality is particularly troublesome because it substantially inflates the chi-square statistic and creates upward bias in critical values for determining coefficient significance. These assumptions will be tested using options available in EQS.

Once the assumptions have been satisfied at acceptable levels, the results will be examined for any offending estimates such as negative error variances, large standard errors, etc. Once it is established that the data meet the assumptions and there are no offending estimates, overall model fit will be assessed by examining goodness-of-fit measures. Goodness of fit is a measure of the correspondence of the actual or observed input (covariance or correlation) matrix with that predicted from the proposed model. Finally, the statistical significance and direction of the paths will be examined and interpreted in light of the hypothesized causal relationships.

Interpreting and modifying the model. Once the model is deemed acceptable, modifications to the model may have to be made to improve its fit further, based on theoretical justification. Modification indices will be examined to improve model fit.

Indirect Effects and Two-Group Analysis

Two additional steps in this analysis will involve examination of significant indirect effects and differences between groups. In this case the two groups used are the industrialized country group (I) and the developing country group (D).

Indirect effects are important for interpretation purposes. For example, PRICEREG affects GBLSALES indirectly through R&DEXPD and INNOVAT. EQS is able to decompose the total effect into direct and indirect effects and provide significance estimates for both.

A second useful feature of EQS used in this study is the analysis of multiple groups to test for significant differences in parameters between two or more groups of interest. In this case, the sample of twenty-seven countries will be divided into two groups, one group consisting of industrialized countries and the other group consisting of developing countries. This will be done to examine if there are significant differences in the relationships between variables for the two groups and whether the models developed fit the two groups equally well, as indicated by the goodness-of-fit indices. Figures 3.3a and 3.3b illustrate the EQS models and structural equations used in the program for the global innovation and the global diffusion models respectively.

FIGURE 3.3a. The EQS Model for Global Innovation

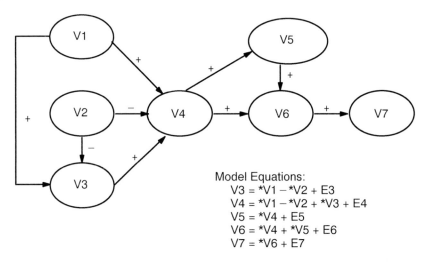

Model Equations:
V3 = *V1 − *V2 + E3
V4 = *V1 − *V2 + *V3 + E4
V5 = *V4 + E5
V6 = *V4 + *V5 + E6
V7 = *V6 + E7

FIGURE 3.3b. The EQS Model for Global Diffusion

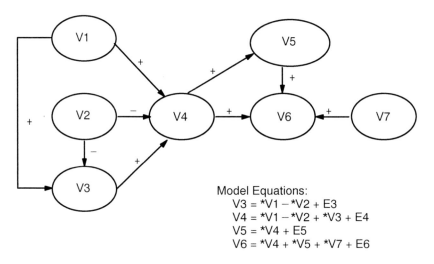

Model Equations:
V3 = *V1 − *V2 + E3
V4 = *V1 − *V2 + *V3 + E4
V5 = *V4 + E5
V6 = *V4 + *V5 + *V7 + E6

Chapter 4

Results

This chapter is divided into five sections. First, results from the analysis of the global innovation models are discussed. Second, results of the two-group analysis, that is, analysis of the differences between the industrialized nations (I) versus the developing nations (D) are discussed. Third, significant indirect effects on innovation and global sales are discussed. Fourth, the results from the global diffusion model are presented. Finally, some concluding comments are offered.

GLOBAL INNOVATION MODEL—RESULTS

A total of thirty-two path models were run using EQS to analyze the factors affecting innovation in the global pharmaceutical industry for the entire sample of industrialized plus developing (I + D) countries. The overall results are illustrated in Figures 4.1 through 4.8. Appendix A contains the tables showing the standardized path coefficients, t-values, standard errors, and the fit indices for the thirty-two runs. All of the individual runs of the model showed a good fit with the hypothesized model. The goodness-of-fit indices varied from 0.998 to 1.000. The chi-square statistic was also indicative of a good fit to the hypothesized model. The results of the individual hypotheses are discussed below.

Effect of GNP, Price Regulation, and Market Size on Innovation

H1: GNP → MKTSIZE

It was hypothesized that countries with a higher GNP/capita would have a larger market size for pharmaceuticals. More than

70 percent of all pharmaceuticals are sold in developed market economies. The developing countries account for less than a fifth of the sales, with the remainder being consumed in East European countries and the former Soviet republics (Ballance, Pogany, and Forstner, 1992). Spending on pharmaceuticals in the developed market economies has been rising. Average pharmaceutical consumption as a percentage of per capita GDP rose from 0.65 in 1975 to 0.95 in 1990. No similar increases have occurred in developing countries. In fact, the share of per capita GDP spent on pharmaceuticals has actually declined in many of the poorer countries (Ballance, Pogany, and Forstner, 1992).

Another factor that affects the market size in the industrialized countries is the demographic characteristics of the population. As the population of a country ages, the need for drugs grows. For the industrialized countries, it is estimated that by the year 2015, over 40 percent of the population will be over forty-five years old. In comparison, only 25 percent of the developing countries' population will be over forty-five years of age by 2015. Public expenditures on health care in the industrialized countries are also higher as compared to the developing countries.

As Figure 4.1 illustrates, the relationship between GNP and MKTSIZE was found to be significant and positive as expected.

H2: GNP → R&DEXPD

According to the technology gap theory of development (Fagerberg, 1987; Posner, 1961; Gomulka, 1971; Cornwall, 1976), there is a close correlation between level of economic development of a nation (measured as GNP or GDP per capita) and level of technological development measured using R&D statistics.

It was therefore hypothesized that countries with a higher GNP/capita would be associated with a more research-intensive pharmaceutical industry reflected in terms of dollar expenditures on pharmaceutical research and development by the respective country's industry. For example, for the period 1980 through 1983, one study estimated that the developed country industries accounted for 96 percent of global R&D expenditure on pharmaceuticals whereas the rest of the world accounted for just 4 percent of global research expenses (Redwood, 1988). The U.S. pharmaceutical industry's total

R&D expenditure was estimated to be $7.3 billion in 1989 (USITC, 1991).

As Figure 4.1 illustrates, the relationship between GNP and R&DEXPD was found to be significant and positive as expected.

FIGURE 4.1. Effect of GNP, Price Regulation, and Market Size on Innovation

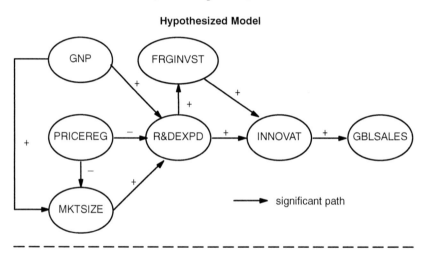

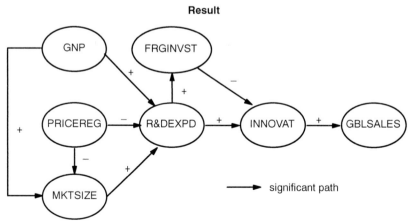

H3: PRICEREG → MKTSIZE

It was hypothesized that the extent of price controls on pharmaceuticals would be negatively related to market size for pharmaceuticals for a country.

In the USITC study, price was found to be inversely related to demand, and price elasticities of -1.12 and -1.28 were found, suggesting that if the price (in real terms) of pharmaceutical products decreases by 1 percent, the quantity demanded of those products would increase by 1.12 to 1.28 percent (USITC, 1991). The United States' large market for pharmaceuticals is in a large part due to the freedom in pricing that manufacturers enjoy. A recent report by the Council on Competitiveness (1991) emphasized freedom from price control as one of three major factors important for continued competitiveness of the U.S. industry.

As Figure 4.1 illustrates, the relationship between PRICEREG and MKTSIZE was found to be significant and negative as expected.

H4: PRICEREG → R&DEXPD

It was hypothesized that the extent of price controls on pharmaceuticals would be negatively related to pharmaceutical R&D expenditure for a country.

Pharmaceutical industries in countries with higher prices have more revenues to reinvest in R&D and have generally well-established and stronger R&D programs as compared to industries with lower-priced products (*European Chemical News,* 1989; Redwood, 1991; USITC, 1991).

Price controls in France have been held responsible for the weak domestic industry. In France, much of the cost of drugs for individual patients is reimbursed by the country's social security fund. Since French governments reportedly have kept drug prices artificially low and the industry has traditionally been dependent on its home market for a large share of its revenues, the flow of research funds to companies has been reduced (*Chemical Marketing Reporter,* 1992a).

As the figure illustrates, the relationship between PRICEREG and R&DEXPD was found to be significant and negative as expected.

H5: MKTSIZE → R&DEXPD

It was hypothesized that the larger the market size for pharmaceuticals for a country, the greater will be its share of global expenditure on pharmaceutical R&D.

Pharmaceutical industries in countries with larger markets have more revenues to reinvest in R&D and have generally well-established and stronger R&D programs compared to industries located in countries with a smaller market size (Parker, 1984; Pradhan, 1983; USITC, 1991).

As mentioned earlier, developed-country industries (having larger country markets) accounted for 96 percent of global R&D expenditure on pharmaceuticals, whereas the rest of the world accounted for just 4 percent of global research expenses in the period from 1980 to 1983 (Redwood, 1988). Among the developed countries, for example, in the period from 1980 to 1983, the United States and Japan were the two largest country markets for pharmaceuticals and simultaneously the top two spenders on pharmaceutical R&D (Redwood, 1988).

As Figure 4.1 illustrates, the relationship between MKTSIZE and R&DEXPD was found to be significant and positive as expected.

H6: R&DEXPD → FRGINVST

It was hypothesized that the greater the expenditure by a country's pharmaceutical industry on R&D, the greater will be the extent of foreign investment by the industry.

This is because companies look to recoup their investments by seeking new markets. Also, the more research intensive the company, the greater is its propensity to take risks and venture into foreign markets. It is also generally the case that high-technology industries are more multinational in nature (Porter, 1990; Dosi and Soete, 1991; Niosi and Faucher, 1991).

One study (Ballance, Pogany, and Forstner, 1992) examined the correlation between R&D expenditures and pharmaceutical exports for seventeen industrialized countries and found the rank correlation to be positive and statistically significant. The relationship was also examined at the company level and was found to be significant. Therefore, substantial research expenditures apparently provide the basis for a pharmaceutical industry's international success as reflected in the large share of sales in foreign markets.

As Figure 4.1 illustrates, the relationship between R&DEXPD and FRGINVST was found to be significant and positive as expected.

H7: R&DEXPD → INNOVAT

It was hypothesized that the greater the expenditure by a country's pharmaceutical industry on R&D, the greater will be its success in originating new chemical entities; in other words, higher R&D expenditures will lead to greater R&D productivity (Franko, 1989).

The study carried out by the U.S. International Trade Commission examined the determinants of national competitiveness in pharmaceuticals comparing the industry in the United States, Western Europe, and Japan using a sample of twenty multinational firms. The study found a significant relationship between R&D commitment and NCE origination (USITC, 1991). The researchers concluded that "pharmaceutical firms must make a considerable commitment to research and development, both in terms of the size of their R&D budget and R&D staff to remain competitive" (p. 6-5).

As the figure illustrates, the relationship between R&DEXPD and INNOVAT was found to be significant and positive as expected.

H8: FRGINVST → INNOVAT

It was hypothesized that the greater the extent of foreign investment (both exports and FDI) by a country's industry, the greater will be the number of NCEs originated by industry. This is because companies that invest abroad are able to exploit the pool of research talents of another country. For example, the Swiss companies in the early 1980s spent almost 40 percent of their total research funds abroad (Dunning, 1988). American member firms of the Pharmaceutical Manufacturers Association spent about 20 percent of their combined R&D budget in 1980 outside the United States.

Also, with respect to this particular study, INNOVAT represents not only the number of NCEs originated by a country's pharmaceutical industry in the period from 1990 to 1994 but also those NCEs that were approved for marketing either at home or abroad. A higher degree of foreign investment should therefore facilitate getting market approval quicker than a lower degree of foreign investment and hence familiarity with foreign markets.

An additional factor that motivates locating R&D facilities abroad is that many products have to be sold worldwide to recoup their development costs, and clinical studies conducted in the host country ensure speedier approval for marketing of the product.

However, as Figure 4.1 indicates, the relationship between FRGINVST and INNOVAT was found to be significant but negative. Prior studies done with respect to other industries have examined the relationship between degree of internationalization and MNE performance measured as profit-to-sales ratio or some other performance measure (Hymer, 1960; Franko, 1987; Grant, 1987; Thomas and Grant, 1987). These studies reported a positive relationship between foreign investment and performance.

However, a study done by Geringer and Beamish (1989) using a sample of 200 MNEs, consisting of the 100 largest firms from the United States and Europe, found that as the extent of foreign investment increased, performance also increased—but it then peaked and exhibited a downward trend. The authors concluded that there is some critical "internationalization threshold" for the companies, and that the relationship between degree of internationalization and performance is more complex than previously imagined.

Several explanations are possible for this phenomenon. As firms encompass increasingly broad geographic markets, the costs associated with geographic dispersion begin escalating, thus eroding performance (in this study, innovative success). With respect to the pharmaceutical industry, in the recent past most foreign investment has taken place in the form of licensing or joint venture arrangements for the purposes of market access rather than FDI or investment in foreign R&D laboratories by the multinationals. This could explain why increased foreign penetration may not necessarily result in greater success with originating NCEs.

H9: INNOVAT → GBLSALES

It was hypothesized that the greater the number of NCEs originated by a country's industry, the greater will be its share of global pharmaceutical sales.

The relationship between technological innovation and performance has been found to be true of all high-technology industries (Rugman, 1985; Porter, 1990; Niosi, 1991). Dozens of studies in econometrics, industrial organization economics, and corporate strategy reveal a significant positive relationship between various indicators of R&D performance/R&D commitment, and performance indicators such as world market share or firm sales growth.

Also, according to the technology growth theory, technology is the principal driving force of the growth of industrialized countries; therefore by extension it should also drive the growth of the individual industrial firms based in those countries (Schumpeter, 1934; Denison, 1967; Carre, Dubois, and Malinvaud, 1975; Harberger, 1984).

According to Grabowski (1989), a leading authority on pharmaceutical innovation and competitiveness, "competition in the multinational pharmaceutical industry centers around the discovery and development of important new drug therapies" (p. 27). The USITC study also found a significant positive relationship between number of R&D drugs and global market share of a firm (USITC 1991, pp. 5-6).

As Figure 4.1 illustrates, the relationship between INNOVAT and GBLSALES was found to be significant and positive as expected.

Effect of GNP, Price Regulation, and Industry Focus on Innovation

H10: GNP → INDFOCUS

It was hypothesized that there is no significant relationship between the level of economic development (GNP) of a country and the extent of concentration or focus of its pharmaceutical industry on pharmaceuticals.

There is no evidence to suggest that richer country industries are any less diversified or more diversified than poorer country industries. In general, European pharmaceutical firms are more highly diversified than American and Japanese firms. This pattern of concentration rather than diversification has historical roots rather than any relation to GNP. American and Japanese firms were mainly pharmacy based or pharmaceutical in origin, whereas many European firms came into the industry through chemicals and dyestuffs (Redwood, 1988).

However, as Figure 4.2 illustrates, the relationship between GNP and INDFOCUS was found to be significant and negative. A possible explanation for this result is that when both industrialized and developing countries are included in the analysis, the relationship between GNP and INDFOCUS becomes significant, since developing country pharmaceutical industries are generally less diversified compared to the industrialized country industries. For the industrialized group the average percentage of sales that was due to pharmaceuticals in this sample was 63 percent, whereas for the developing country group, the average percentage of sales that was due to pharmaceuticals was 83 percent.

H11: PRICEREG → INDFOCUS

It was hypothesized that the greater the level of price control on pharmaceuticals, the lower would be the concentration of the industry on pharmaceuticals.

The more favorable the conditions for pharmaceutical profitability, the greater would be the focus on sales of pharmaceutical products. However, as the figure illustrates, the relationship between PRICEREG and INDFOCUS was found to be positive instead of negative as expected.

Again, this result is possible due to the nature of the sample—consisting of both developing and industrialized countries—and the large differences in the nature of the industries between the two. The developing countries have a higher degree of price control but are also more focused on pharmaceuticals compared to the industrialized country group, simply because of the nature of the economic

FIGURE 4.2. Effect of GNP, Price Regulation, and Industry Focus on Innovation

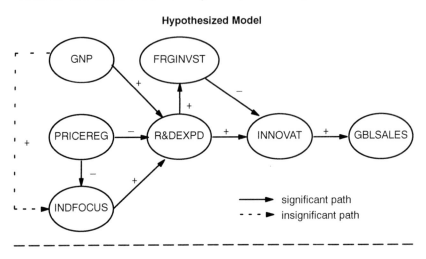

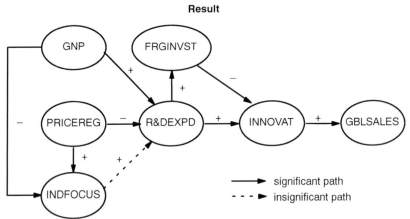

and political conditions, thus resulting in the positive relationship between **PRICEREG** and **INDFOCUS**.

H12: INDFOCUS → R&DEXPD

It was hypothesized that the greater the focus on pharmaceuticals by a country's industry, the greater would be the expenditures on pharmaceutical research and development. This is because pharmaceutical industries are generally found to increase their concentration on pharmaceutical-related products when the climate for pharmaceutical profitability is favorable. Since R&D is an important aspect of pharmaceutical profitability, by extension a higher focus should result in higher R&D investment. As Figure 4.2 illustrates, the relationship was positive but insignificant.

The insignificance of the relationship could again be attributed to the effect of the developing countries in the sample, i.e., a high focus but low R&D expenditure compared to the industrialized countries.

Effect of GNP, Price Regulation, and Industry Growth on Innovation

H13: GNP → INDGRWTH

It was hypothesized that there is a positive but insignificant relationship between GNP and industry growth (measured as average percentage change in sales from 1990 to 1994). However, as Figure 4.3 illustrates, the relationship between GNP and INDGRWTH was found to be negative but not significant.

This could be because the pharmaceutical industry in the developing countries has been growing at a much faster rate (particularly in the recent past) than the industry in the industrialized countries, which is fairly stable and well established. For example, the average percentage change in sales for the developing country sample in this study was 13 percent, whereas for the industrialized countries the change was 12 percent.

H14: PRICEREG → INDGRWTH

It was hypothesized that the greater the level of price control on pharmaceuticals, the lower would be the average growth in pharmaceutical industry sales for the country.

There is anecdotal evidence to suggest that industry sales growth is affected by level of price controls. However, as Figure 4.3 illustrates, the relationship was found to be positive although insignificant.

FIGURE 4.3. Effect of GNP, Price Regulation, and Industry Growth on Innovation

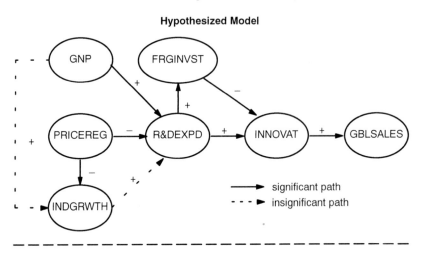

Hypothesized Model

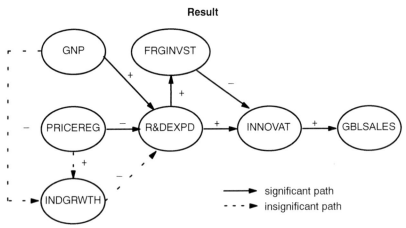

Result

This could be due to a couple of reasons. First, countries that have a very profitable industry have also been the ones to be subjected to greater price controls in the recent past, thus accounting for the positive direction of the relationship. This is especially true in the case of industrialized countries. The two-group analysis discussed later in the chapter reveals this to be the case.

Second, as explained above, developing country industries are the ones experiencing greater growth but also have a higher degree of price control compared to the industrialized countries, thus resulting in the positive direction of the relationship. When the developing countries are analyzed separately as a group the relationship is negative as hypothesized.

H15: INDGRWTH → R&DEXPD

It was hypothesized that growth in industry sales would be positively but insignificantly related to R&D expenditures. The link between corporate R&D and firm sales growth has been tested in the industrial organization literature both across and within industries. Results have typically shown an association between measures of R&D input and firm growth (Franko, 1989; Scherer, 1976; Mansfield, 1968; Leonard, 1971; Jarrell, 1983; Comanor, 1986). These studies, however, used mononational U.S. samples, so the relationship has not been tested for a worldwide international sample.

As Figure 4.3 illustrates, the relationship was found to be negative and insignificant. Again, the effect of the developing countries in the sample is the possible culprit, that is, the high industry growth rates in recent years coupled with the lower R&D expenditures in the developing country group when compared to the industrialized group, giving us the negative relationship between INDGRWTH and R&DEXPD. Later in the two-group analysis it will be seen that the relationship is positive for the industrialized country group alone.

Effect of GNP, Price Regulation, and Industry Concentration on Innovation

H16: GNP → INDCONC

It was hypothesized that there is an insignificant relationship between a country's GNP/capita and the concentration of the pharmaceutical industry in that country.

This was based on prior literature which showed little difference in the concentration ratios of the industry for countries with varying ranges of economic development. For example, Redwood (1988) examined the market share held by the top twenty firms for thirteen industrialized and thirteen developing countries using 1984 data. He found no significant pattern in the relationship between concentration and level of development and concluded that this was because the leading multinational firms have a commanding position in both groups of nations.

However, as Figure 4.4 illustrates, GNP was found to be *significantly* inversely related to INDCONC, implying that the more developed countries had a less concentrated industry structure.

Examination of more recent data on concentration ratios reveals that the degree of oligopoly power is more pronounced in developing countries than in the industrialized countries. For example, the twenty-five-firm concentration ratios using 1988 data were compared for industrialized versus developed country groups by Ballance, Pogany, and Forstner (1992). The average twenty-five-firm concentration ratio for developing countries was sixty-three compared to fifty-seven for the industrialized group.

Possible reasons for this difference are that the domestic industry in the poorer countries is relatively weak, along with the incomplete regulatory system in these countries that allows abuse of market power by the multinationals. The implications of this are worrying for policymakers and consumers in the developing world.

H17: PRICEREG → INDCONC

It was hypothesized that there is no significant relationship between degree of price control and industry concentration for a country.

This is because there is a lack of any research study regarding the pharmaceutical industry that examines the above relationship even with single country samples, let alone multicountry samples such as this one. Although the industrial organization and economics literature generally points to the negative effects of regulation on market competition (Kamien and Schwartz, 1982; Rothwell and Zegveld, 1981), there was insufficient anecdotal or empirical evidence regarding the pharmaceutical industry that the relationship would be significant.

As Figure 4.4 illustrates, PRICEREG had a positive but insignificant impact on INDCONC.

FIGURE 4.4. Effect of GNP, Price Regulation, and Industry Concentration on Innovation

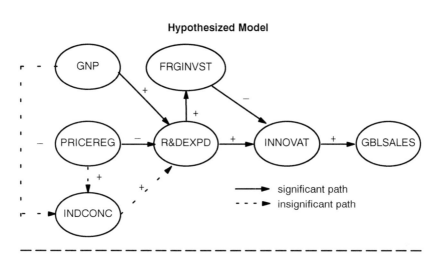

Hypothesized Model

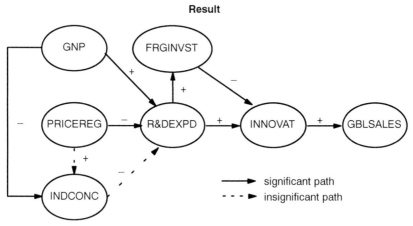

Result

H18: INDCONC → R&DEXPD

The relationship between market structure and indicators of innovation has been statistically tested by industrial organization economists.

Schumpeter's hypothesis that a "competitive oligopoly" is most conducive to innovation provided the impetus for several studies in this area (Niosi, 1991). Other researchers argued a similar position, being that since research is generally not a profitable activity, only sufficiently large firms can carry out research knowing they will benefit from its results (Villard, 1958; Phillips, 1956; Kamien and Schwartz, 1970; Loury, 1979).

Experts in the pharmaceutical industry also generally concede to the oligopolistic characteristics of the industry due to its research-intensive nature (Grabowski, 1976; Schwartzman, 1976). Based on the above, it was therefore hypothesized that INDCONC would be positively related to R&DEXPD.

As Figure 4.4 illustrates, the relationship was found to be negative although insignificant. However, as will be discussed later, the two-group analysis revealed a positive relationship between IND-CONC and R&DEXPD. That is, when the industrialized and developing country samples are tested separately, the relationship is in the direction expected. Therefore, pooling the two groups results in confounding effects for certain variables.

Effect of Population, Approval Time, and Market Size on Innovation

H19: POP → MKTSIZE

Generally, the larger the population, the greater the market size for pharmaceuticals. As expected the relationship was positive and significant.

H20: POP → R&DEXPD

Larger populations should result in larger market size (as explained above) and, consequently, greater revenues to invest in R&D. It was therefore hypothesized that more populated countries would be associated with greater levels of expenditure on pharmaceutical R&D. As the figure shows, the relationship was positive and significant as expected.

H21: APPTIME → MKTSIZE

A high degree of regulation should have a negative effect on market size. That is, the greater the stringency of the approval procedure for marketing new pharmaceuticals, the longer it will take for the new product to reach the market—thus reducing market availability of new products and therefore reducing potential market size. Therefore, a negative relationship was hypothesized between APPTIME and MKTSIZE. However, as Figure 4.5 illustrates, APPTIME was positively associated with MKTSIZE, although the path was statistically insignificant.

Most studies in the pharmaceutical industry literature have examined the relation of APPTIME to innovation rate. The only study examining the APPTIME → MKTSIZE relationship is by Parker (1984), where he ranked countries by regulatory tightness and examined a series of rank correlations between the former and various indicators of market size. All correlations were significant and positive. This is because countries that have large markets for pharmaceuticals are also the ones that are most stringent in their approval procedures for marketing of new pharmaceuticals, thus possibly explaining the above result.

H22: APPTIME → R&DEXPD

Delays in the marketing approval process can reduce a product's effective patent life, thus reducing the period in which a company can recoup its R&D expenditures. Studies on pharmaceutical innovation indicate the negative effects of long approval times on the rate of innovation (Grabowski and Vernon, 1976; Grabowski, Vernon, and Thomas, 1978; Wardell, 1973, 1975).

APPTIME should therefore have a negative effect on R&D EXPD. However, as Figure 4.5 illustrates, the relationship was positive but statistically insignificant. Again, the confounding effect of the sample was suspected. That is, industrialized countries have longer approval times but also larger R&D expenditures compared to developing countries, resulting in the positive relationship. When two-group analysis was done, the effect was negative but insignificant for the two groups (I&D).

FIGURE 4.5. Effect of Population, Approval Time, and Market Size on Innovation

Hypothesized Model

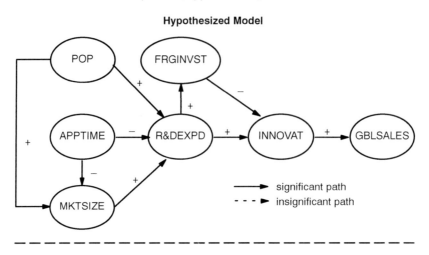

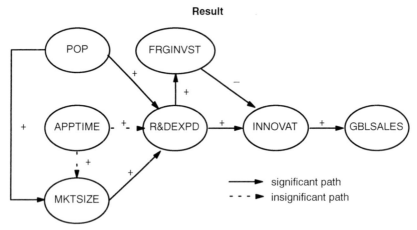

Effect of Population, Approval Time, and Industry Focus on Innovation

H23: POP → INDFOCUS

It was hypothesized that the larger the population, the greater would be the focus of the industry on pharmaceuticals due to the larger market for pharmaceuticals. The relationship was found to be positive and significant as expected.

H24: APPTIME → INDFOCUS

There is little in the literature to suggest that regulatory stringency has a direct effect on the level of industry focus or diversification. Therefore it was hypothesized that the effect would be negative but statistically insignificant. As Figure 4.6 illustrates, the hypothesis was confirmed.

Effect of Population, Approval Time, and Industry Growth on Innovation

H25: POP → INDGRWTH

It was hypothesized that a larger population size would have a positive effect on growth in industry sales; however, the effect would not be statistically significant. As Figure 4.7 illustrates, the above hypothesis was confirmed.

H26: APPTIME → INDGRWTH

As mentioned earlier, the relationship between APPTIME and rate of innovation has been the subject of examination by most researchers. One can speculate that a higher rate of innovation would fuel higher sales growth and, therefore, approval times should affect INDGRWTH.

Based on the above, it was hypothesized that APPTIME is negatively related to INDGRWTH. However, as Figure 4.8 illustrates, the relationship was found to be positive but insignificant.

This may be because approval times for most countries have remained fairly stable, at least for the past decade, rendering it difficult to isolate the effect of changes in regulatory approval times on changes in sales growth. A longer time frame would be needed to isolate this effect.

FIGURE 4.6. Effect of Population, Approval Time, and Industry Focus on Innovation

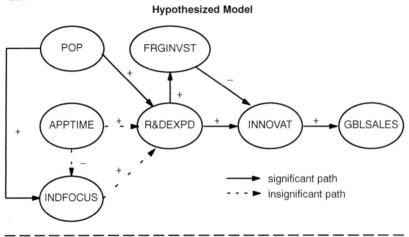

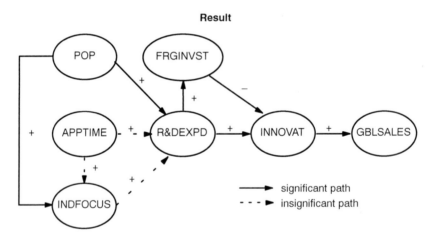

Effect of Population, Approval Time, Industry Concentration, and Foreign Commitment on Innovation

H27: POP → INDCONC

Theoretically, in a competitive industry, a larger market size should stimulate more entries into the industry. Therefore, if a large

FIGURE 4.7. Effect of Population, Approval Time, and Industry Growth on Innovation

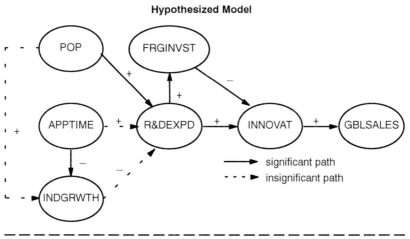

Hypothesized Model

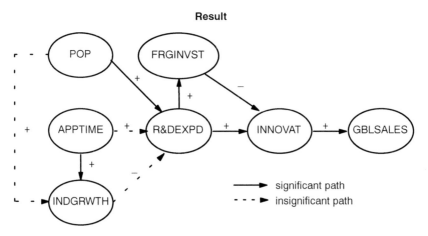

Result

population translates to a larger potential market, then INDCONC should be lower when POP is higher.

However, no firm conclusions are possible due to the oligopolistic nature of the global pharmaceutical industry in individual countries. It was therefore hypothesized that there is a negative but insignificant relationship between POP and INDCONC. As Figure 4.8 illustrates, the relationship is positive but insignificant.

FIGURE 4.8. Effect of Population, Approval Time, Industry Concentration, and Foreign Commitment on Innovation

Hypothesized Model

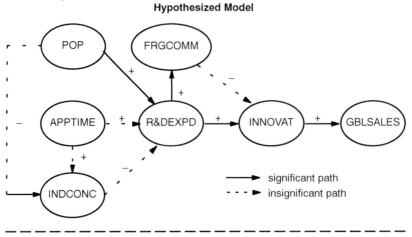

Result

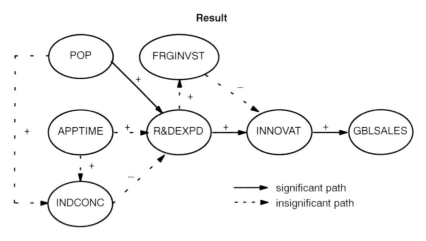

The positive direction of the relationship could be due to the inclusion of the developing countries in the sample that have a much larger population but also show higher INDCONC compared to industrialized countries. Two-group analysis (discussed later in this section) reveals a negative relationship between POP and IND-CONC for the industrialized countries, as would be expected.

H28: APPTIME → INDCONC

As mentioned earlier, the relationship between APPTIME and rate of innovation has been the subject of frequent examination by most researchers. One can speculate that more stringent approval procedures would deter firms from entering the industry, therefore resulting in greater industry concentration.

No firm conclusions are possible, however, due to the oligopolistic nature of the global pharmaceutical industry in individual countries and the domination of a few multinational firms in most countries. It was therefore hypothesized that there is a positive but insignificant relationship between APPTIME and INDCONC. As the figure illustrates, the relationship is positive but insignificant.

H29: R&DEXPD → FRGCOMM

It was hypothesized that the level of investment in research and development by a country's pharmaceutical industry would be positively associated with the level of commitment to investment in overseas markets. This is because firms need to recoup their R&D investment in as many ways as possible, one of which is greater sales in foreign markets. As the figure shows, the relationship was found to be positive but insignificant. This can be explained on the basis of home market size. Countries whose industries show a high percentage of foreign sales are those with relatively smaller domestic markets.

For example, industries in countries such as Switzerland, Belgium, Denmark, and so on, derive more than 80 percent of their pharmaceutical sales from nondomestic sources because of their smaller home market size. Countries such as the United States and Japan on the other hand show a much smaller degree of foreign commitment due to their huge home markets.

Thus R&D investment does impact the absolute level of foreign investment (see H6) but not necessarily the level of foreign commitment expressed as share of foreign to total sales.

H30: FRGCOMM → INNOVAT

Despite the multinational character of the industry, most of the basic research is still done in the laboratories of the home country.

A higher level of commitment to foreign markets may not, therefore, necessarily result in greater innovative success. In fact, it could have the opposite effect of diverting attention and resources away from basic research to the increased complexity of managing diverse foreign investments. This was found to be the case in H8 (FRGINVST → INNOVAT).

Another factor is the knowledge and familiarity required with the local FDA approval procedures. Most FDA agencies are likely to approve home country applications faster than applications from foreign companies. INNOVAT in this study represents not only the number of NCEs originated by a country's industry but those NCEs that were approved for marketing either at home or abroad. INNOVAT is likely to be higher when most of the NCEs have been originated and approved for marketing in the same country.

Therefore, it was hypothesized that the relationship between FRGCOMM and INNOVAT would be negative but insignificant. Figure 4.8 shows that the hypothesis was confirmed.

GROUP DIFFERENCES—INDUSTRIALIZED AND DEVELOPING COUNTRIES

The sample of twenty-seven countries was divided into two groups. The countries were classified based on Ballance, Pogany, and Forstner's (1992) classification of countries' pharmaceutical industries. The above researchers grouped countries into four groups (A, B, C, and D), based on the technological sophistication of a country's pharmaceutical industry.[1] The country sample in this study was divided into two groups. Group 1 consisted of Group A countries which were mostly industrialized countries (fifteen in all), and Group 2 consisted of Group B and C countries which were mostly developing countries (twelve in all).

The research question of interest here was: is there a difference in the direction and magnitude of influence of various factors that affect innovation, and hence global competitiveness of the pharmaceutical industry of industrialized nations versus that of the developing nations? Again, thirty-two runs on EQS were carried out with the two groups (tables in Appendix A show the results of the thirty-two program runs).

Table 4.1 lists the paths that were significantly different in the two groups. No specific hypotheses for the two-group analysis were developed since this analysis was exploratory in nature due to lack of similar studies in the literature. The paths for which significant differences were found are discussed below.

GNP → MKTSIZE

The gross national product of a country was found to have a significant positive effect on the market size for pharmaceuticals in the industrialized (I) country group. The relationship was insignificant and negative for the developing (D) country group.

This effect seen for the D group can be explained based on the nature of the health care systems in developing countries. First, poorer developing countries spend a greater proportion of their health care budget on pharmaceuticals (especially the third world countries). Thus, the GNP of a developing country may not be a significant factor in determining market size for pharmaceuticals and may well have a negative effect by way of reducing public health expenditures on pharmaceuticals.

TABLE 4.1. Significant Path Differences Between Industrialized (I) and Developing (D) Country Groups

Path	Significance		Direction	
	I	D	I	D
1. GNP → MKTSIZE	Significant	Insignificant	+	−
2. PRICEREG → R&DEXPD	Significant	Insignificant	−	+
3. MKTSIZE → R&DEXPD	Significant	Insignificant	+	−
4. R&DEXPD → INNOVAT	Significant	Insignificant	+	−
5. FRGINVST → INNOVAT	Significant	Insignificant	−	+
6. INNOVAT → GBLSALES	Significant	Insignificant	+	−
7. PRICEREG → INDCONC	Significant	Insignificant	−	−
8. INDCONC → R&DEXPD	Insignificant	Significant	+	+
9. POP → R&DEXPD	Significant	Insignificant	+	−
10. POP → INDFOCUS	Significant	Insignificant	+	+

PRICEREG → R&DEXPD

The level of price controls on pharmaceuticals had a significant negative effect on expenditures on R&D for the I group but the effect was opposite and insignificant for the D group.

This difference is not surprising in view of the fact that pharmaceutical industries in the industrialized countries are heavily research based and their R&D activities would be more sensitive to future profits and therefore pricing regulation. The pharmaceutical industries in the D group are not based on basic research but concentrate heavily on the manufacture of bulk pharmaceuticals and formulations.

The positive (although insignificant) effect observed for the D group could be due to the presence of Group B-type countries that do have a small research base but are also characterized by greater price regulation.

MKTSIZE → R&DEXPD

A larger market for pharmaceuticals had a strong positive effect on innovation investment, that is, R&D expenditures for the I group; the effect was insignificant and negative for the D group.

This result is indicative of the vast difference in the nature of the pharmaceutical industries in the two groups. As explained earlier, the research-based industry in the industrialized countries will be more sensitive to the underlying factors affecting innovation compared to the industry in the developing countries. Since research is a costly and time-consuming process, market size would greatly affect the level of investment in research.

However, a larger market in developing countries does not necessarily mean a higher investment in innovation and may even reduce the investment in R&D as shown by the result. This may be for several reasons. For example, the absence of patent protection in countries in the D group reduces the incentive for spending on R&D for new drug development. A larger market size in these countries would therefore result in greater concentration of efforts in other activities such as improving manufacturing technology for basic chemicals, acquiring distribution channels, greater foreign exporting of bulk formulations, and so on.

R&DEXPD → INNOVAT

The level of investment in innovation has a strong positive effect on innovative success for the I-group countries; the effect is insignificant and negative for the D group. This implies that investment in R&D is more efficiently and productively utilized in the I group than in the D group. The difference is not surprising (as previously explained) due to the research-based nature of the industry in the I group.

The negative effect of R&D expenditure on innovation for the D group was not statistically significant but is important for interpretation purposes, since it indicates either inability to utilize R&D resources efficiently or that R&D resources in countries in the D group are more efficiently utilized in other activities rather than basic research.

FRGINVST → INNOVAT

The level of foreign investment had a strong negative effect on innovation for the I group; the effect was insignificant and positive for the D group.

The pharmaceutical industry of industrialized countries is multinational in character. Recent cost-containment pressures in national markets have driven the industry further to explore alternative markets abroad. However, as explained in the discussion of the above path for the overall group analysis, overexpansion into foreign markets can result in diversion of resources from basic research to managerial activities, thus affecting innovative success (INNOVAT).

The same is not true for developing country industries, since their extent of foreign involvement is restricted to exports of mainly bulk formulations and generic pharmaceuticals. Besides, the industry is not primarily research based in this group. Thus the insignificant effect of FRGINVST on INNOVAT for the D group is not surprising.

INNOVAT → GBLSALES

The number of new drugs developed (INNOVAT) has a strong positive effect on global competitiveness (GBLSALES) of the pharmaceutical industries in the I group. The effect is insignificant and negative for the D group.

This result has serious implications for developing countries and challenges the generalized assumption in the literature that *all* countries (regardless of their stage of economic development) need to invest in innovation for global competitiveness.

The negative and insignificant relationship between INNOVAT and GBLSALES for the D group implies that there are other avenues by which developing country industries can be globally competitive and that, at least for now, ability to develop NCEs is not one of them. The prospects and strategies that developing countries should follow are discussed in greater detail in Chapter 5.

PRICEREG → INDCONC

Price regulation had a strong negative effect on extent of industry concentration for the I group countries; the effect was insignificant for the D group.

The strong significant effect of regulation on market structure in industrialized countries versus the weak effect of regulation in the developing countries is expected, since the markets for pharmaceuticals are larger and more competitive in the developed economies. However, the negative effect of PRICEREG is surprising since greater price pressure should result in higher concentration in the industry.

This effect is plausible, however, due to the presence of competition from the generic pharmaceutical industry. Greater price control on patented drugs (as is normally the case in I-group countries) will induce more generic firms to enter the industry, thus possibly lowering overall concentration ratios for the industry.

INDCONC → R&DEXPD

Industry concentration levels had a significant positive effect on the level of R&D expenditures for the D-group countries; the effect was insignificant for the I group.

In recent years, the pharmaceutical industry in the developing countries has been experiencing increasing concentration ratios.

This upward trend has been more pronounced for the developing countries than the industrialized countries where the ratio has remained fairly stable. Pharmaceutical industries in the developing world have been increasing spending on research and, as we have seen earlier, the oligopolistic nature of the industry is especially favorable for greater research spending.

Thus, the level of concentration in the developing countries that are still dominated by a handful of multinationals has a more significant effect on level of R&D expenditures than seen in the industrialized countries, where there is not as much variation with respect to concentration ratios in the sample.

POP → R&DEXPD

Population size has a strong positive effect on research spending in the industry for the industrialized countries; the effect is insignificant and negative for the developing countries.

A larger population for an industrialized country translates into a larger market size for pharmaceuticals; the same is not true for developing countries, as the more populated developing countries are characterized by low purchasing power. A larger market size should therefore be associated with greater spending on R&D for the I-group countries, which is the effect observed in this case.

Therefore, pharmaceutical industries in large industrialized countries such as the United States are at an advantage, compared to industries in small industrialized countries with a small home market, such as Switzerland.

POP → INDFOCUS

Population size was significantly associated with level of industry focus for the I-group countries; the effect was insignificant for the D group.

As explained above, a larger population in industrialized countries implies a larger home market. The larger the market for pharmaceuticals, the greater should be the focus of the industry on pharmaceutical products rather than on nonpharmaceuticals. This also explains why the pharmaceutical industry in countries with larger home markets, such as the United States and Japan, have less diversified pharmaceutical industries than countries with more diversified pharmaceutical industries, such as Switzerland or Belgium, due to their small home markets.

Overall Evaluation of the Differences Between I and D Groups

In general, the global innovation model showed a better fit for the industrialized group than for the developing country group in terms of the number of significant paths found. This result is interesting and has serious implications for further research with respect to economic development. Most research done on industrialized country samples generalizes the findings to developing countries, because data on developing countries is scarce. These study results show that generalization of models and findings used for industrialized countries cannot be universally applied.

According to Lall (1990), a leading expert on economic development and an advisor to the OECD, developed economies have often tried to apply the same neoclassical principles to developing countries with negative results. The structure of incentives, factor markets, policies, institution, and infrastructure in the developing countries is far too different to be subjected to the same economic policies as those applied to the industrialized economies. In addition, differing social, economic, political, and cultural traditions cast their own influence on the direction and pace of capability development.

A study by Fagerberg (1987) tested the technology gap models using a sample of OECD and non-OECD countries, where he examined the relationship between technology variables such as growth in innovative activity and economic development of the country. He found the models "better suited" for industrialized countries than the developing countries. He concluded that the developing countries have followed a separate way of development and that if differences in growth between these countries had to be explained, a much more detailed analysis of "economic, social and institutional structures needed to be carried out" (p. 64).

SIGNIFICANT INDIRECT EFFECTS ON INNOVATION AND GLOBAL COMPETITIVENESS

Several constructs had significant indirect effects on innovation and global sales (global competitiveness).

As seen in Figure 4.9, pharmaceutical innovation (INNOVAT) was affected by a country's macroeconomic environment (GNP and POP); the regulatory environment (PRICEREG); and its market/industry structure (MKTSIZE).

Both GNP and POP had significant positive effects on innovation, implying that pharmaceutical industries based/located in countries with a higher GNP/capita and a larger population are more successful at developing NCEs.

PRICEREG had a significant negative indirect effect on innovation as expected, that is, the less favorable the regulatory environment in a country for its pharmaceutical industry, the lower is the innovative success of the industry.

The home market size (MKTSIZE) of a country had a significant positive effect on innovation; that is, industries based in countries

FIGURE 4.9. Significant Indirect Effects

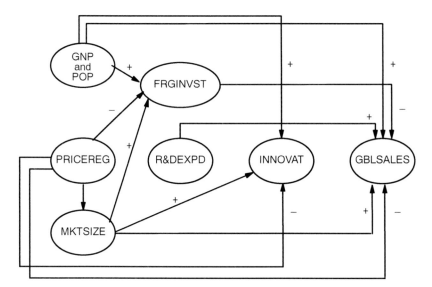

with a large market potential for pharmaceuticals are more success-ful at developing and introducing innovative new drugs (NCEs).

Global competitiveness (GBLSALES) was also indirectly affected by a country's economic environment (GNP and POP); regulatory environment (PRICEREG); market/industry structure (MKTSIZE); investment in innovation (R&DEXPD); and the level of foreign investment (FRGINVST).

In general, pharmaceutical industries based in countries with a higher gross national product per capita, larger population, lower price regulation, larger market size, higher investment in research and development, and moderate foreign investment were more glob-ally competitive.

GLOBAL DIFFUSION MODEL—RESULTS

As discussed in Chapter 3, the global diffusion model had several constructs in common with the global innovation model, since several of the factors that affect supply also affect demand. In all, seven paths were of interest in the global diffusion model as listed in Table 3.3b. To test for the seven hypothesized paths, twelve separate runs on EQS were carried out. Appendix B shows the results for the global diffusion model.

The global diffusion model was tested only for the industrialized group of countries since few developing countries in the sample were recipients of new drug introductions. Thus results of the global diffu-sion model apply only to the industrialized group of countries. Figure 4.10 shows the results of the global diffusion analysis.

H1: INDFOCUS → MKTPOT

It was hypothesized that a higher industry focus on pharmaceuti-cal products would be positively associated with market potential. As the figure illustrates, this hypothesis was confirmed. The under-lying causal effects on market potential are important when analyz-ing diffusion models, since larger markets should attract greater diffusion of new products. Thus foreign pharmaceutical firms can benefit by choosing countries that show a higher overall industry focus on pharmaceuticals when introducing new drugs.

FIGURE 4.10. Global Diffusion Model

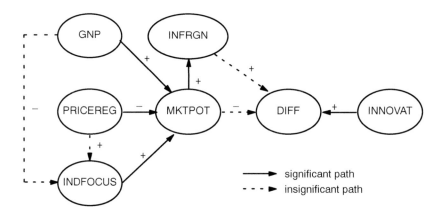

A higher host country focus on pharmaceuticals can have other positive effects, such as greater familiarity of regulatory agencies with new drug development procedures, pricing mechanisms, and other public policy issues related to pharmaceuticals.

H2: INDGRWTH → MKTPOT

Industry growth was found to have an insignificant effect on market potential. This is because most industrialized countries have had fairly stable growth rates in recent years without much variation among the countries in this respect. Therefore, market potential is not significantly affected by growth in sales of the pharmaceutical industry. However, even though the relationship is insignificant, positive growth reflects a healthy industry and therefore a viable market. Pharmaceutical firms will in general be better off introducing their products into countries where the pharmaceutical industry shows positive percentage changes in annual sales.

H3: INDCONC → MKTPOT

Level of industry concentration was insignificantly related to market potential. It was hypothesized that countries with industries characterized by greater concentration would be associated with smaller market size for pharmaceuticals. However, the relationship between industry concentration and market size is not established in the literature. Due to the supposedly oligopolistic nature of the industry, it is difficult to predict the effect of concentration on market potential. Therefore, foreign pharmaceutical companies looking to introduce products in other countries should not be deterred by concentration ratios of the industry in those countries, since there still could be a large untapped market out there for investment.

H4: MKTPOT →INFRGN

A larger market potential was hypothesized to have a significant positive effect on inbound foreign investment. As shown in the figure, this hypothesis was confirmed. Larger markets are bound to attract greater foreign investment in the industry. The United States is a particularly attractive market and has attracted a great deal of foreign investment by Swiss, British, and other Western European pharmaceutical firms.

H5: MKTPOT →DIFF

It was hypothesized that market potential would have a significant positive effect on the number of NCEs introduced into the country (DIFF). However as the figure illustrates, the relationship was insignificant. This could be explained on the basis of Parker's study (1984) in which he found that larger markets did not necessarily attract more new drug introductions than smaller markets. He speculated that such an effect was possible because most large country markets are also the ones with the most stringent regulatory procedures; thus the effect of regulation canceled out the effect of market size.

In this study DIFF represents the number of new drugs launched for the first time in any country. Generally, pharmaceutical companies choose those countries whose regulatory procedures they are most familiar with for first launch of a new drug. Usually this is the home country, although there can be exceptions such as the United

States, where in recent years more U.S.-based companies are choosing other countries for first launch, due to the unusually long approval periods in the United States.

Once the drug has achieved market success in the country of first launch, then it is generally easier for the firm to obtain approval for marketing in other, more attractive (larger market size) countries. Therefore, a higher MKTPOT may not necessarily be positively related to DIFF in this case.

H6: INFRGN → DIFF

It was hypothesized that the greater the incoming foreign investment in the country's pharmaceutical industry, the higher will be the number of NCEs introduced into the country. This is because firms would invest in countries that offer attractive returns in terms of large market size, easier approval procedures, or to exploit local talent in research or other areas. Some of these factors would favor NCE introduction into the country's markets.

As Figure 4.10 shows, the relationship was positive but insignificant. As explained in the previous hypothesis, a firm's choice of the country for first launch of an NCE depends on a complex set of factors, especially a combination of various regulatory policies such as patent protection policies, product liability issues, acceptance of foreign clinical data, and so on.

In this study, only two regulatory variables were used, namely price control and approval time for marketing of NCE. Although it would have been desirable to test as many regulatory variables as possible, constraints on data availability and other resources made this difficult.

Also, in the past, most foreign investment by pharmaceutical companies has increasingly been in the form of informal alliance arrangements, such as licensing or other marketing agreements for gaining market access for drugs that have already been approved elsewhere. Therefore, the extent of inbound foreign investment may lead to a greater number of first time NCE launches, but the effect may be insignificant due to the nature of foreign investment.

H7: INNOVAT → DIFF

It was hypothesized that a higher number of NCEs developed by a country's pharmaceutical industry (INNOVAT) would be associated with higher number of NCEs first launched into the country (DIFF). This is because, as explained previously, most firms choose the home country or the country in which the NCE was developed (originating country) as the country for first launch. This is due to the ease in getting marketing approval from the local regulatory agency.

It could also be explained on the basis of demand creating supply. A higher perceived demand for a product would lead a firm to develop the product for that market in which it is located, thus making it more likely that the originating country would be the recipient country for the NCE.

As Figure 4.10 illustrates, INNOVAT had a strong positive effect on DIFF, confirming the relationship between supply and demand factors of innovation.

CONCLUSIONS

The results of the global innovation model analysis provide interesting insights into the factors affecting innovation in the pharmaceutical industry. A country's economic, regulatory and market/industry environment has significant effects on the innovativeness of its pharmaceutical industry. The results also indicate that greater innovation overall leads to greater global competitiveness. Analysis of the GIM model also reveals the need for analyzing the industrialized and developing countries separately.

Two-group analysis of the industrialized and developing countries reveals significant differences between the determinants of innovation for the two groups. In general, the GIM shows a better fit for the industrialized countries and a poor fit for the developing country group. The managerial and public policy implications of the above results are discussed in Chapter 5.

Global innovation and global competitiveness are significantly affected indirectly by a number of factors. In general, pharmaceutical industries based in countries with a higher gross national product per capita, larger population, lower price regulation, larger market size, higher investment in research and development, and moderate foreign investment were more globally competitive.

Results of the global diffusion model analysis revealed that the level of global innovation had a far greater impact on the extent of diffusion of NCEs into a country than the market potential or level of inbound foreign investment for the country. This relationship confirms the theory that supply and demand factors of innovation strongly affect each other. The result also implies that factors that impact global innovation can also impact global diffusion.

Table 4.2 provides an overall summary of the results for the three groups analyzed (I + D; I; and D) for the global innovation model.

TABLE 4.2. Summary of Results—Global Innovation Analysis

Path Relationships	Significance of Paths			Direction		
	I+D	I	D	I+D	I	D
1. Economic Env → Mkt/Industry Structure						
GNP → Mkt size	sig	sig	insig	+	+	−
GNP → Industry focus	sig	insig	insig	−	−	−
GNP → Industry growth	insig	insig	insig	−	−	+
GNP → Industry conc	sig	insig	insig	−	+	+
Population → Mkt size	sig	sig	sig	+	+	+
Population → Industry focus	sig	sig	insig	+	+	+
Population → Industry growth	insig	insig	insig	+	+	+
Population → Industry conc	insig	insig	insig	+	−	+
2. Economic Env → Innovation Investment						
GNP → R&D Expend	sig	sig	sig	+	+	+
Population → R&D Expend	sig	sig	insig	+	+	−
3. Regulatory Env → Mkt/Industry Structure						
Price control → Mkt size	sig	insig	insig	−	−	−
Price control → Industry focus	sig	sig	insig	+	+	+
Price control → Industry growth	insig	insig	insig	+	+	−
Price control → Industry conc	insig	sig	insig	+	−	−
Approval time → Mkt size	insig	insig	insig	+	+	−
Approval time → Industry focus	insig	insig	insig	+	+	−
Approval time → Industry growth	insig	insig	insig	+	+	−
Approval time → Industry conc	insig	insig	insig	+	+	+
4. Regulation → Innovation Investment						
Price control → R&D Expend	sig	sig	insig	−	−	+
Approval time → R&D Expend	insig	insig	insig	+	−	−

TABLE 4.2 (*continued*)

5. Mkt/Industry Structure → Innovation Investment							
Mkt size → R&D Expend	sig	sig	insig	+	+	−	
Industry focus → R&D Expend	insig	insig	insig	+	+	−	
Industry growth → R&D Expend	insig	insig	insig	−	+	−	
Industry cone → R&D Expend	insig	insig	sig	−	+	+	
6. Innovation Investment → Foreign Investment							
R&D Expend → frgn invst	sig	sig	sig	+	+	+	
R&D Expend → frgn comm	insig	insig	insig	+	−	+	
7. Innovation Invst → Global Innovation							
R&D Expend → Innovat	sig	sig	insig	+	+	−	
8. Foreign Invst → Global Innovation							
Frgn invst → innovat	sig	sig	insig	−	−	+	
Frgn comm → Innovat	insig	sig	insig	−	−	+	
9. Global Innovation → Global Sales							
Innovat → Gbl Sales	sig	sig	insig	+	+	−	

Chapter 5

Conclusions

This chapter has five sections. The first section provides a summary of the results of the study. The second section discusses the managerial and public policy implications of the study results for industrialized and developing countries. The third section examines the theoretical, empirical, and methodological contributions of the study. Next, some study limitations are discussed, and finally, future prospects for the global pharmaceutical industry are examined.

SUMMARY OF RESULTS

Determinants of Global Innovation

One of the research objectives of the study was: Which country factors stimulate or inhibit a nation's pharmaceutical industry to be globally innovative? The main findings as a result of the analyses of the global innovation models follow:

1. The economic environment of a country has a significant impact on the market and industry structure of its pharmaceutical industry as well as on pharmaceutical innovation investment.
2. The regulatory environment of a country has a significant effect on pharmaceutical market and industry structure as well as on pharmaceutical innovation investment.
3. A large market size for pharmaceuticals is associated with greater investment in pharmaceutical innovation.
4. Increases in innovation investment lead to increased global innovation.

5. Only moderate levels of foreign investment lead to increased global innovation. A high level of foreign diversification has a negative effect on global innovation.
6. Global innovation is positively associated with global competitiveness, that is, the greater the number of NCEs developed, the greater is the global market share of the country's industry.
7. Global competitiveness of the pharmaceutical industry was significantly indirectly affected by its national economic, regulatory, and market/industry environments.

Of the economic variables, GNP had a greater effect on market and industry structure variables than POP. Market size, industry focus, and industry concentration were all affected by economic factors. Industry growth was the only aspect of market/industry structure that was not influenced. Both GNP and POP also affected R&DEXPD.

Of the regulatory variables, only PRICEREG was significant. APPTIME did not have a significant effect on any of the dependent variables. Pricing regulation had a strong negative effect on market size. It also affected industry focus and lowered innovation investment.

Market size was the only significant variable of all the market/industry structure variables to have an effect on innovation investment. A larger pharmaceutical market size had the effect of increasing investment in innovation.

Higher levels of innovation investment seemed to drive levels of total foreign investment and global innovation higher. Finally, global innovation was a strong determinant of global competitiveness.

Global Innovation Factors for Industrialized versus Developing Country Industries

The main findings as a result of analyzing the two groups (industrialized and developing) of countries follow:

1. The economic environment of industrialized countries had a greater impact on the market and industry structure of the pharmaceutical industry, as well as on pharmaceutical innovation investment, compared to developing countries.

2. The regulatory environment of industrialized countries had a more significant effect on pharmaceutical market and industry structure, as well as on pharmaceutical innovation investment, compared to developing countries.
3. A large market size for pharmaceuticals is associated with greater investment in pharmaceutical innovation in the case of industrialized country firms; the effect is negative and not significant for developing country firms.
4. Increases in innovation investment lead to increased global innovation for the industrialized country industries; the effect is negative and not significant for the developing country industries.
5. A high level of foreign investment has a negative effect on global innovation for industrialized countries; the effect is opposite but insignificant for developing country industries.
6. Global innovation drives global competitiveness of industrialized country firms, but has a negative although insignificant effect on developing country competitiveness.
7. Global innovation in the pharmaceutical industry in industrialized countries is significantly *indirectly* affected by its national economic, regulatory, and market/industry environments; no significant indirect effects are obtained for the developing country industries.

In general, the global innovation model had a better fit for the I group in terms of the number of significant paths than for the D group. More significantly, perhaps, none of the direct causal variables of global innovation and global competitive advantage had any significant effects for the developing country group. This implies that factors other than those related to innovation are responsible for global competitive advantage of the developing country pharmaceutical industries. A second important implication of the above findings is that results for industrialized country markets cannot be generalized to developing country markets, both for managerial and especially for public policy purposes.

Determinants of Global Diffusion

A second research objective of the study was: Which country factors stimulate or inhibit diffusion of pharmaceutical innovations into a country's markets? The global diffusion model was analyzed only for the I group; therefore the results apply only to industrialized countries. The main findings follow:

1. The nation's economic, regulatory, and market/industry environment all had a significant effect on the market potential for diffusion of NCEs.
2. Greater market potential for pharmaceutical diffusion led to increased inbound foreign investment in a country's pharmaceutical industry.
3. Global diffusion of pharmaceuticals was not directly affected by market potential or inbound foreign investment, but was strongly affected by the level of global innovation.

With respect to the economic environment, only GNP had a significant effect on market potential for diffusion. The effect of population size was absent. Of the regulatory variables, only PRICEREG was an important factor affecting market potential; APPTIME had no effect. Of the market/industry structure variables, industry focus was the only factor significantly affecting market potential.

Contrary to expectations, global innovation was a more significant explanatory variable of global diffusion than market potential and inbound foreign investment. That is, countries characterized by a highly innovative pharmaceutical industry were also more likely to be recipients of pharmaceutical innovations. That is, NCE originating countries are also the destination countries for NCEs.

IMPLICATIONS OF STUDY RESULTS

Managerial Implications

Although the study examines factors affecting competitiveness at the national level and the industry level, the results have implications at the firm level since national-level policies can affect firm strategy and vice versa. Managerial implications of study results for firms from industrialized countries and developing countries are discussed separately due to significant differences found between the two groups.

Strategy Implications for Industrialized Country MNCs

As discussed in Chapter 2 in the review of literature, the global strategic management literature was reviewed to draw implications for pharmaceutical MNCs from the study results. Three streams of thought in the literature were found to be applicable to this study: (1) core competencies, (2) comparative advantage-based competitive advantage, and (3) collaborate to compete.

Core competencies. As defined earlier, core competencies are "the collective learning in the organization, especially the coordination of diverse production skills and integration of multiple streams of technology" (Prahalad and Hamel, 1990, p. 82).

According to most experts in global strategy and competitiveness, firms must possess some core competency that is difficult for competitors to imitate in order to have sustained competitive advantage.

The results of this study show that ability to innovate is causally related to global sales or global competitiveness in the pharmaceutical industry. Further, the environment for innovation is affected by the home country's economic, regulatory, and market/industry environments. Thus the key to competitive advantage for industrialized country pharmaceutical firms will be in developing core competencies in R&D as well as being able to strategically manage their R&D programs with respect to changing economic, regulatory, and market/industry conditions of the countries in which they operate.

A good example is the Japanese MNCs. In response to a stagnating economy, increasing price pressures from the Japanese government, and greater foreign competition in the home markets, several Japanese pharmaceutical firms have in the recent past invested heavily in R&D research units in the United States and abroad, along with marketing agreements with major U.S. and European multinational companies involving licensing and co-marketing agreements (Yoshikawa, 1989).

Several U.S. multinationals are now focusing their R&D efforts on only a few therapeutic categories, with more research being disease-based rather than symptom-based. This is in response to the increasing costs of research and the increasing regulatory and competitive pressure such as competition from generic manufacturers (*Financial World*, 1989).

A second area of core competency in the pharmaceutical industry is in marketing (Bogner and Thomas, 1992). Analysis of the global diffusion model revealed that the market potential for diffusion is significantly affected by a nation's economic, regulatory, and market/industry environments. Thus selection of international markets for investment or introduction of new products should be undertaken only after a careful evaluation of the above environmental factors. Firms can develop core competencies with respect to being able to identify changes in environmental conditions for investment purposes.

The dynamic environment in the European Community offers an especially appropriate illustration of this problem. Due to the unification of the European Community markets and the effort toward harmonizing the various environments, pharmaceutical firms in the European Community have been faced with great uncertainties with respect to future market conditions. Firms that can strategically manage their marketing programs in coordination with these changing environmental conditions will be at a distinct competitive advantage in the future. An example to illustrate this is the alliances developed by small local companies in the European Community to attract foreign multinationals for licensing purposes. For example, Derma Alliance is an alliance of dermatological companies comprising small local firms from Norway, the United Kingdom, Germany, Spain, and France, formed in direct response to the changing EC environment. The idea of this alliance is to offer big multinationals development, regulatory, and marketing help with their licensed products (Longman 1994). By licensing a product to one of the alliance members, a licensor can acquire local partners in all major European markets and speed its time to market.

Comparative advantage-based competitive advantage. This concept implies the design of international strategies based on the interplay between the comparative advantages of countries and the competitive advantages of firms (Kogut, 1985).

Comparative advantage, sometimes referred to as location-specific advantage, arises out of the differences in factor costs across national markets. Thus a firm can gain cost or other advantages by configuring its value chain so that its activities are located in those countries that have the lowest cost for a particular factor. National differences can also arise in the markets for firm outputs. Some of these differences arise from varying consumer tastes and preferences, as well as different institutional arrangements that affect the output markets (Kochhar and Hitt, 1995).

Competitive advantage, sometimes referred to as firm-specific advantage, influences what activities and technologies along the value-added chain a firm should concentrate its resources in, that is, the core competency of the firm.

Industrialized countries differ with respect to the environmental conditions of their markets for the global pharmaceutical industry. Differences in national economic, regulatory, and market/industry environments can be sources of comparative advantage to industrialized MNCs.

For example, with respect to regulatory environment, firms based in the United States have a comparative advantage as they can benefit from the freedom from price controls on pharmaceuticals. PRICEREG was found to be a significant variable affecting both innovation investment and the market potential for diffusion. At the same time, APPTIME—time taken by the regulatory agencies to approve a new drug for marketing—was found to have little effect on the innovation environment as well as on the market potential for diffusion. Thus companies need be less cautious of national differences with respect to this regulatory aspect in their strategic location decisions.

Population (POP), for example, was found to be a significant determinant of both market size (MKTSIZE) and R&D expenditure (R&DEXPD). Industrialized countries with large populations could be a source of comparative advantage to firms based in those countries. The large populations in the United States and the United Kingdom, compared to countries such as Belgium or Switzerland, are definite sources of comparative advantage to pharmaceutical firms looking for large markets.

Collaborate to compete. In recent years, several experts have studied the effectiveness of alliances in international business and found them to be an important weapon of competitive advantage in the global competitive arena (Hamel, Doz, and Prahalad, 1989; Harrigan, 1987; Ohmae, 1989). According to Hamel and colleagues, "it takes so much money to develop new products and to penetrate new markets, that few companies can go it alone in every situation" (p. 133).

According to Shan and Hamilton (1991), such international cooperative ventures provide a firm with access to country-specific advantages embedded in its partners. In the opinion of the above researchers, "international cooperative relationships may be viewed as a vehicle to tap into the comparative advantages of countries" (p. 419). In an empirical study of a sample of domestic and international cooperative relationships of Japanese firms in the biotechnology industry, Shan and Hamilton found country-specific advantages to be a significant variable in explaining differences between cooperative relationships with partners of different countries.

The case for collaboration is particularly strong in the global pharmaceutical industry in the present environment. The combined effects of patent erosion, new research methodology, competition from generics, and a rise in the real costs of R&D are forcing companies into mergers, acquisitions, and alliances. The case for mergers and acquisitions is stronger when attention turns to marketing. Larger operating units are a logical way to cut marketing costs and gain access to new buyers. Few drug producers (particularly European ones) have distribution systems in place in both Japan and the United States, the world's two biggest markets.

Japanese MNCs have been especially active in taking advantage of country-specific differences in their choice of collaborations. For example, results of the global innovation and diffusion models reveal the effect of national environmental differences on the markets for developing and introducing NCEs. Firms based in these varying national environments have these effects embedded in them to a certain extent and are better able to deal with the environments in which they are located.

Japanese firms, by entering into strategic alliances with U.S. and Western European firms, manage to get access to registration and development systems in these countries. For example, Takeda, a major Japanese multinational, established a joint venture in the United States with Abbott Laboratories to develop and market ethical drugs. Takeda also has ties with firms in Germany, France, and Italy, and funds research at Harvard and Tulane Universities (*Business Week*, 1990).

Merck, the U.S.-based multinational, formed an alliance with Sigma Tau of Italy in 1982 to co-market a number of products in Italy (USITC, 1991). Italy's market is highly nationalistic and foreign firms need to develop a close relationship with governmental agencies to obtain more timely approval and attractive pricing. This is possible only through marketing alliances with domestic companies. Merck and Sigma Tau have also entered into a research joint venture agreement, with the Italian company seeking to tap into the comparative advantage in research of the U.S.-based company.

Strategy Implications for Developing Country MNCs

As discussed in Chapter 4, the analysis of the global innovation model revealed a poor fit with respect to developing country pharmaceutical industries. In addition, several significant differences as well as opposite effects were found between the industrialized country group and the developing country group.

This result has important implications. Most research done on industrialized country samples generalizes the findings to developing countries since data on developing countries is scarce. The results of this study show that such generalizations cannot be made.

The negative and insignificant relationship between INNOVAT and GBLSALES for the D group implies that innovation is not a significant determinant of global sales for developing country firms and that there may be other sources of competitive advantage that developing country MNCs can employ. Some recommendations with respect to the strategies that such MNCs can employ are discussed using a framework similar to that above.

Core competencies. The pharmaceutical industry in the developing countries consists mostly of reproductive firms (Ballance, Pogany, and Forstner, 1992). These firms are mostly locally owned, subsidiaries of multinationals, or joint ventures between indigenous and foreign companies. In several of these countries, the firms do no more than produce the finished product from imported inputs.

However, there are certain core competencies that developing country firms can cultivate in order to compete in the global marketplace. The example of Indian pharmaceutical firms is illustrative.

Like many other developing countries, India recognizes patents only for processes. Some of its companies specialize in developing new chemical processes, yielding drugs that are identical to those produced (at much greater expense) by multinationals. The Indian firms begin by selling their new products domestically; later, they scale up operations to cut manufacturing costs. The foreign markets that they select as targets are countries that recognize process patents but not patents on the product itself. By the time the companies are ready to export, they can often sell the drugs at less than a tenth of the price charged by competitors in industrialized countries (Ballance, Pogany, and Forstner, 1992; Narayana, 1984).

The growth of generic markets and the many drugs that will soon come off patent mean that a greater portion of the world's markets could soon be open to producers in developing countries.

Some of the newly industrializing countries such as Singapore, South Korea, and Taiwan are aggressively targeting the biotechnology market for the future (Howe, 1992, 1993). These countries have created technology centers, offered tax incentives, and tried to improve basic science research in order to develop more competent scientists. Korea has been able to compete on high-volume, low-cost products throughout the Southeast Asian region.

Comparative advantage-based competitive advantage. Developing countries differ significantly among themselves with respect to their national economic, regulatory, and market/industry environments for pharmaceuticals. That is, countries differ with respect to their comparative advantages. As explained previously, such differences can be exploited for purposes of gaining competitive advantage by multinational firms.

For example, Hong Kong is looking into developing a partnership with China, offering its business skills and tapping China's scientific expertise, low wages, and plentiful natural resources. The Hong Kong Institute of Biotechnology has partnered with the Chinese

Academy of Sciences to identify marketable compounds from traditional Chinese remedies (Howe, 1993). Hong Kong may then use the expertise it gains to launch its own industry, and as a result become competitive in the future.

Third-world MNCs can take advantage of the booming economies of the NICs and their growing markets for pharmaceuticals. For example, Singapore has attracted new material production, formulation, and packaging plants because of the attractive incentives offered by the Singapore government. Singapore is poised to become the medical treatment and distribution center for the Southeast Asian region.

Collaborate to compete. For developing country MNCs, competing via participation in joint ventures or alliances is a particularly useful mode for entering the global market. Since most firms from such countries are small, with insufficient research and production resources, collaboration can provide the means to pool resources and acquire access to new markets.

Most Western pharmaceutical companies, for example, choose to enter developing country markets through joint ventures. Developing country firms can gain important technological know-how from the more advanced multinationals in return for their marketing expertise and familiarity with local governmental agencies.

China, for example, is establishing growing links with firms from industrialized countries that are interested in developing retail and OTC products from traditional Chinese herbal remedies. Some foreign participants hope to make use of Chinese research on biological agents that they could convert into drugs. Other arrangements call for Chinese scientists to conduct the research and for the collaborator to develop the products. Later, the Chinese are expected to test the prototypes in research facilities provided by the overseas partner (Ballance, Pogany, and Forstner, 1992).

Public Policy Implications

The pharmaceutical industry is unique in that it is one of the few industries in which, in almost all countries, the government plays an important role and takes a keen interest in industry operations. Because the industry has such social importance, the government sees itself as a major regulating force and acts by formulating a variety of policies affecting the industry in critical ways.

Public Policy Implications for Industrialized Countries

The results of the study reveal that a country's economic, regulatory, and market/industry environment have a significant impact on the factors that directly affect global competitiveness. Further, these environments are also found to exert significant indirect effects on global competitiveness in the pharmaceutical industry.

With respect to the economic environment, GNP was found to be a significant variable affecting market size, industry focus, and industry concentration. It was also found to impact investment in innovation. Thus, industrialized country governments need to evaluate the nation's economic environment before taking policy measures with respect to the pharmaceutical industry. A robust economy seems necessary for a thriving industry.

Population size was also a significant factor affecting both market size and industry focus. The large industrialized countries with significant populations should take advantage of this in promoting the pharmaceutical industry further.

With respect to the regulatory environment, price control was the only significant factor affecting competitiveness. It had a significant negative effect on market size and R&D investment for innovation. It also had a significant indirect negative effect on both innovation and global sales. Further, it also had a significant negative impact on the market potential for diffusion of new drugs.

Industrialized countries need to develop creative means of price control such that incentives for industrial innovation are not affected and health care is accessible to all at the same time. The United Kingdom is one country that has been successful in this attempt. It uses a program called PPRS. This is a voluntary program and is intended to maintain price levels that allow for a "reasonable return on capital," to ensure that prices of pharmaceutical products are not raised arbitrarily, and to limit the cost of drugs to the National Health Service (NHS). The PPRS is credited with having increased investment in the British pharmaceutical industry (Taggart, 1993).

In contrast, the price control program used in Germany is expected to negatively impact innovation in the future. The program utilizes the concept of therapeutic clustering, and has reportedly resulted in a 25 to 40 percent decrease in pharmaceutical prices in Germany. Therapeutic clustering, or the grouping of drug products for similar indications for reimbursement at similar price levels by either health insurance plans or national health systems, regardless of whether the products are patent protected, is expected to exacerbate the impact of cost-containment efforts.

Pricing controls have also been enacted in almost all of the European Community countries. The implementation of price controls in the European Community has resulted in price differentiation in the individual countries, which has, in turn, resulted in increased parallel trade. The undercutting in price that results from parallel trade results in decreases in revenue, which could in turn have a potentially negative impact on R&D.

With respect to market/industry environment, market size was the most important factor affecting R&D expenditures as well as outbound foreign investment. A large home market size promoted greater investment in innovation and had a significant indirect effect on global competitiveness. Thus, industrialized country governments need to maintain market demand in the home country by implementing appropriate policies that have the effect of increasing pharmaceutical market size. One of the means by which this can be achieved has already been discussed; namely, restricting policies that implement stringent price controls.

Innovation investment or R&D expenditure had a direct effect on global innovation (number of NCEs developed), which in turn was a strong explanatory variable of global sales (global competitiveness). Policies in industrialized countries should therefore be geared to increase industrial investment in innovation. National funding agencies such as the NIH in the United States have been important sources of R&D funding for the industry. Japan reportedly has nineteen different tax incentive systems to encourage technological innovation, including an R&D tax credit similar to that in the United States. Federal government support for medical research in the United States continues to exceed funds allocated by other national governments (USITC, 1991).

Global innovation was also the most important determinant of global diffusion. This implies that factors that encourage global innovation will also encourage global diffusion. To be frequent first-time recipients of new drug discoveries (NCEs) is obviously an important social goal for all industrialized countries. Introduction of NCEs into the market also has the effect of increasing industry competition and thus driving innovation. Thus, all of the previously mentioned policy issues relevant for industrial innovation are also relevant for increasing diffusion of NCEs into the country.

In sum, public policies in industrialized country markets must be geared toward increasing GNP, increasing market demand for pharmaceuticals, restricting price control measures, and increasing investment in R&D in order to promote global competitiveness of its pharmaceutical industry.

Public Policy Implications for Developing Countries

As discussed earlier, policies that work for industrialized countries are assumed to be universally applicable for all developing and underdeveloped countries to achieve the same level of economic development.

Lall (1990), advisor to the OECD, believes that such conventional approaches lead to wrong policy responses. For example, the World Bank's structural adjustment policy recommendations for industry in developing countries have little directly to say about the time lag between policy changes and supply response, human resource development, or the needs of institution building. They barely differentiate among countries' different levels of development.

In most studies related to technology and economic growth, "technology" is taken to be freely available to all countries and, within countries, to all firms. To the extent that technology lags are admitted, developing countries are taken to receive all relevant improvements from developed country innovators; there is no problem in assimilating the transferred technology; no adaptations are required, and so forth.

The results of this study show that the causal variables for global competitive advantage in the pharmaceutical industry not only have opposite effects for developing country industries but also that these effects overall may not be significant in explaining the determinants of competitiveness. This has significant implications for public policymakers and consultants to the pharmaceutical industries in developing countries.

Policymakers in developing countries need to focus on the following aspects to improve the position of the firms both nationally and internationally:

1. Improve and strengthen the scientific base for development and production of traditional medicine and household remedies.
2. Invest in development of repackaging and formulation plants.
3. Advance development and production of bulk drugs, including immunologicals and antibiotics.
4. Establish regulations relating to domestic and foreign corporate ventures and the importation of foreign drugs, intermediates, and know-how.
5. Review pricing and patent protection policies for increasing market attractiveness for foreign investment.
6. Promote exports of pharmaceutical preparations and encourage international collaborations with both developing and industrialized country firms.

Public policymakers are often guilty of being too enamored of gadgetry and high technology, thus distorting the pattern of investment in health care supplies and pharmaceuticals. Governments in these countries need to appreciate that they cannot quickly achieve the same level of sophisticated technology as the United States or Japan. Developing countries will have to make the best use of what is currently available, because advanced innovation is beyond their means or not as important as other needs.

LIMITATIONS OF THE STUDY

The major limitation is with respect to the nature of international data used in the study. Differences in accounting terms and techniques exist. The definition of pharmaceutical business is also notoriously varied. Shifts in exchange rates have affected performance; for example, in recent years the Europeans and Japanese have benefited from the depreciation of the dollar. Therefore, some of the data may not be capable of direct comparison. However, maximum effort has been made wherever possible to correct for inconsistencies and ensure the comparability of the data used in this study.

A second limitation is with respect to the time frame used in the study. Data over a four-year period (1990 to 1994) was used. Resource constraints with respect to time available to the researcher for collecting and inputting the data in a usable form prevented use of a longer time frame for the study. However, this is not considered a major limitation but may in fact have been the appropriate time frame to use. This is because a longer time frame would have introduced confounding effects due to the significant changes in the global environment of the pharmaceutical industry taking place in the late 1980s. Availability of a longer time frame would have necessitated splitting the analysis into two time periods to weed out the confounding effects. It would of course be interesting to do a two-period analysis to observe any differences with respect to the effect of the various factors tested.

A third limitation of the study is that it focuses on a single industry—the pharmaceutical industry. Results may not be generalizable to other industries. However, the path models and the variables tested are general enough to be applied to other industries as well. Thus, future research could be done for other industries as well.

Finally, a greater number of regulatory variables need to be tested with respect to their effect on innovation and diffusion of NCEs. Difference between countries with respect to their product liability laws, patent protection legislation, licensing and joint-venture policies, and so on have important effects on the rate of intercountry innovation and diffusion of NCEs. Inclusion of each additional variable to the models used in this study would have greatly increased the complexity of the research design and rendered interpretation of the results difficult.

CONTRIBUTIONS OF THE STUDY

Theoretical Contributions

The present study makes significant theoretical contributions to several streams of literature, namely the literature on national competitiveness, pharmaceutical innovation and diffusion, economic development, and global strategic management.

National competitiveness literature tests theoretical concepts in the theory of comparative advantage, the technology factor theory, Porter's theory of the national diamond of competitiveness, and the role of government in national competitiveness.

Comparative advantages of countries with respect to their economic, regulatory, and market/industry environments are found to be important for competitiveness in the pharmaceutical industry. Technology—the ability to innovate—is found to be a significant factor in global competitive advantage for the pharmaceutical industry. Both factor and demand conditions in Porter's diamond of national competitive advantage were tested empirically with regard to the pharmaceutical industry and found significant.

The debate on the role of government in national competitiveness was tested in this study with respect to a single industry. The regulatory factors were found to significantly affect the determinants of competitiveness.

The theoretical literature on pharmaceutical innovation and diffusion makes a contribution by considering factors beyond just the effect of regulatory variables that most studies in the above literature have examined. This study tests a comprehensive model, considering a variety of supply and demand factors affecting pharmaceutical innovation and diffusion.

The contributions of this study to the theories on economic development are also important. By empirically testing the same model for both industrialized and developing countries, the results show that determinants of competitive advantage vary significantly for the two groups. The results refute the generalized assumption of the technology factor theory that developing countries can simply imitate the industrialized country model of technology and increase their rate of economic growth.

The study results also provide interesting insights for the global strategic management literature. Most importantly, the study points to the importance of national environments and the need for firms to be able to adapt to varying economic, regulatory, and industry environments to be competitive. Most global strategic management research has tended to focus on factors endogenous to the firm and ignored the macro factors affecting firm competitiveness in the global economy (Bolton and Boyacigiller, 1993).

Empirical Contributions

The present study makes significant empirical contributions to the global competitiveness literature on the pharmaceutical industry.

According to the U.S. International Trade Commission report (USITC, 1991), most studies in the previously mentioned literature have focused on U.S. firms, using mononational samples or binational samples at the most. There are just a handful of studies using several country samples focusing on overall factors affecting all countries taken together.

A second shortcoming in the research on global competitiveness in the pharmaceutical industry is that most studies have considered only regulatory factors and excluding additional factors that are as important if not more.

A third weakness in previous research on global competitiveness in the pharmaceutical industry, identified by USITC, is the primary focus on supply-related factors of innovation. Demand-related factors have been ignored, that is, factors affecting demand for pharmaceutical innovations across national markets, which are of great strategic importance (USITC, 1991).

A fourth shortcoming is the predominant focus on the industrialized countries. Admittedly, it is the industrialized country firms that play a major role in the global competition in pharmaceuticals; however, one cannot forget the enormous social importance of the industry and its role in improving quality of life for all humans. Competitiveness issues with respect to the developing countries' pharmaceutical industries deserve more attention and research.

The present study attempts to overcome these limitations as follows:

1. The study utilizes a sample of over 200 firms, representing twenty-seven countries. This is far more than the USITC (1991) study, which used twenty-nine firms representing seven countries for assessing competitiveness.

2. The study examines the effect of several variables in addition to regulatory variables, such as GNP, population size, market size, industry focus, industry concentration, industry growth, foreign investment, foreign commitment, and so on, on pharmaceutical innovation.
3. The study examines both supply-related and demand-related factors affecting global competitiveness in the pharmaceutical industry as recommended in the USITC 1991 report.
4. The study examines both industrialized countries and developing countries, finding significant differences between the two, with crucial managerial and public policy implications for developing countries emerging as a result of the analysis.

Methodological Contributions

This study uses structural equation modeling (SEM) to test the path diagrams developed from the theoretical literature. SEM is an extension of several multivariate techniques and provides a means of dealing with multiple dependence relationships simultaneously while providing statistical efficiency (Hayduk, 1987). To the best of this researcher's knowledge (Agrawal), there are no studies using the above statistical method in the research on pharmaceutical innovation and diffusion. The few empirical studies in this area use regression techniques best.

Managerial and Public Policy contributions

The results of this study make significant contributions with respect to the managerial and public policy literature.

THE GLOBAL PHARMACEUTICAL INDUSTRY ENVIRONMENT IN THE FUTURE

During 1997, downward pressure on pharmaceutical sales and prices continued throughout the year as governments around the world tried various means to tackle the problem of escalating health care costs. Several governments, such as those of France and Spain, also tried to encourage the development of the generics industry in an attempt to bring down prices. Price cuts were on the menu in Belgium and Austria. The Italian government continued to come under fire for its "average European price" mechanism, which industry said had managed to push Italian prices 30 percent below the actual European average. Germany, France, and Switzerland all considered various means to contain prices of pharmaceuticals in 1997. The results of this study show that pricing regulation has a strong negative effect on market size, industry focus, and innovation investment. Innovation investment, in turn, was found to affect global competitiveness. National policymakers should be careful when tackling the problems of pharmaceutical pricing. Continued pressure on prices is expected in the future, which could further erode the innovation potential of the industry.

Several markets and regions attracted attention in 1996 and 1997 as having good growth potential. China is increasingly being viewed as a market that cannot be ignored. Various multinationals set up joint ventures with local companies during the period. Growth forecasts for China project a compound annual growth rate of more than 16 percent by 2001, compared with 6.2 percent for the world pharmaceutical market (*Scrip,* 1998). Various reports predicted great market potential in India, with its population of 950 million, 150 million of whom apparently have purchasing power approaching that of the middle classes in the West. However, price controls and the lack of new patent legislation are still seen as short-term problems. In the developing world, Brazil attracted considerable pharmaceutical investment in 1997. This was partly due to Brazil's new patent legislation, which took effect in May 1997, as well as greater economic stability, growing purchasing power, and price increases for medicines. The Latin American pharmaceutical market in general is expected to grow substantially in the coming years. Expected features of the market include more political stability and patents, more generics, and more managed care and private health care insurance. The markets in the Middle East are also expected to grow. Currently Turkey, Iran, and Israel account for 68 percent of the Middle East market.

The area of research that enjoyed the biggest boom in 1997 was genomics. Genomics, functional genomics, and pharmacogenomics were heralded as the likely sources of an abundance of new targets for therapeutics. Numerous alliances were formed between pharmaceutical companies and those offering various types of sequencing, combinatorial chemistry, or screening expertise.

Strategic alliances in R&D continued at full pace in 1997. Over 100 major collaborations signed included research alliances, licensing agreements, and technology deals. These alliances covered the whole range of R&D activities—from licensing deals covering compounds in late phase development to collaborative research projects to discover human disease-causing genes. The big money was spent on alliances for compounds in the late stages of development. Eli Lilly, Genentech, Warner-Lambert, Merck, and Proctor & Gamble were some of the multinationals actively involved in R&D alliances in 1997. Acquisitions and mergers continued in 1997 with companies trying to consolidate their positions in particular markets.

Macroeconomically, the coming years for the global pharmaceutical industry do not look bright. Only in the United States, and possibly in one or two smaller countries, do the economies look capable of delivering a growth rate for the pharmaceutical sector in excess of 7 percent. The Far East tiger economies are in trouble. Japan is struggling to find its way back to the growth levels achieved in the 1980s and is finding it hard going, so pharmaceutical companies should not look to that source for above-average growth. The member states of the European Union are politically and economically preoccupied with the euro currency issue. Eastern Europe, Latin America, the Middle East, and other global regions will not deliver the strong economic growth needed to boost pharmaceutical companies' expectations.

R&D will have to be more productive. As illustrated by Zantac's example, there is little that a company can do to preserve the revenues and profits of an ex-patent drug. Patent expiry is just that, a loss of monopoly which can only be replaced by a new and better monopoly in the form of a unique compound. Industry leaders claim that the new technologies such as genomics, combinatorial chemistry, computer drug design, and so on are transforming the R&D process from a random exercise to one that is far more predictable and certain. Although this is true in terms of being able to help companies discover more lead compounds, the gamble as to whether the lead compounds will translate into safer, more medically and economically effective medicines is as great as ever. The issue for companies is not that there is a shortage of lead compounds, but which are the right ones to choose for the long and costly haul through the clinical evaluation process. The biotech companies long regarded as the saviors of the pharmaceutical industry are themselves facing an uncertain future at the technical level. With the wealth of gene information pouring out, it is no longer sufficient for a biotech company to specialize in just one gene, say for diabetes, since such exclusivity cannot be sustained. As a result, biotech companies are having to broaden their bases and become more generalized research organizations.

On the regulatory front, the major change in the future is the abolition of national applications for new product marketing approvals in the European Community. Starting in 1998, the only forms of approval will be through the centralized system or the decentralized system. Demands by the pricing authorities for cost-effectiveness data will continue along with increasing pressure on doctors to prescribe generically.

In conclusion, the pharmaceutical companies of the industrialized countries as well as those from the developing countries need to focus on their core competencies; exploit the comparative advantages of countries around the world with respect to differences in their national economic, regulatory, and industry environments; and collaborate strategically with both domestic and international firms in order to compete in the global marketplace.

Appendix A

Global Innovation Models

TABLE A.1. Global Innovation Model

Paths	Overall	Industrialized	Developing
v3,v1	0.190[a]	0.423	-.129
Economic Env →	(0.167)[b]	0.225	.265
Mkt/Ind Structure	1.084[c]	1.725	-.486
v3,v2	-0.365	-0.397	-.030
Regulation →	(0.167)	0.225	.265
Mkt/Ind Structure	-2.087	-1.618	-.113
v4,v1	0.026	0.192	.483
Economic Env →	(0.066)	0.090	.233
Innovation Invst	0.374	1.850	2.208
v4,v2	-0.165	-0.330	.180
Regulation →	(0.070)	0.089	.231
Innovation Invst	-2.128	-3.217	.832
v4,v3	0.856	0.685	-.218
Mkt/Ind Structure →	(0.075)	0.107	.232
Innovation Invst	11.307	6.049	-.995
v5,v4	0.901	0.846	.890
Innovation Invst →	(0.085)	0.167	.120
Foreign Mkt Invst	10.777	5.263	7.319
v6,v4	1.561	1.537	-.885
Innovation Invst →	(0.170)	0.235	.497
Global Innovation	9.310	6.882	-1.672
v6,v5	-0.776	-0.885	.947
Foreign Mkt Invst →	(0.168)	0.226	.504
Global Innovation	-4.627	-3.962	1.790

v7,v6 Global Innovation→ Global Sales	0.896 (0.086) 10.489	0.848 0.164 5.306	−.008 .267 −.031
Fit Indices Chi-square; df p-value BBFI BBNFI CFI	22.16;12 0.046 1.000 1.000 1.000	7.207;12 0.843 1.000 1.000 1.000	13.007;12 .368 1.000 1.000 1.000

a = standardized coefficient, b = standard error, c = t-value

v1 = gnp, v2 = pricereg, v3 = mktsize, v4 = r&dexpd, v5 = frginvst, v6 = innovat, v7 = gblsales

TABLE A.2. Global Innovation Model

Paths	Overall	Industrialized	Developing
v3,v1 Economic Env → Mkt/Ind Structure	-0.336[a] 0.168[b] -1.911[c]	-0.67 0.287 -0.573	-.256 .247 -1.008
v3,v2 Regulation → Mkt/Ind Structure	0.226 0.168 1.287	0.193 0.287 0.664	.181 .247 .714
v4,v1 Economic Env → Innovation Invst	0.241 0.163 1.385	0.552 0.130 3.680	.417 .224 1.980
v4,v2 Regulation → Innovation Invst	-0.511 0.158 -3.044	-0.685 0.131 -4.545	.252 .221 1.217
v4,v3 Mkt/Ind Structure → Innovation Invst	0.147 0.176 0.825	0.418 0.135 2.732	-.372 .234 -1.735
v5,v4 Innovation Invst → Foreign Mkt Invst	0.901 0.084 10.79	0.847 0.166 5.274	.890 .120 7.319
v6,v4 Innovation Invst → Global Innovation	1.561 0.170 9.312	1.538 0.234 6.886	-.885 .497 -1.672
v6,v5 Foreign Mkt Invst → Global Innovation	-0.776 -0.779 -4.627	-0.885 0.226 -3.962	.947 .504 1.790
v7,v6 Global Innovation → Global Sales	0.896 0.904 10.498	0.848 0.164 5.313	-.008 .267 -.031
Fit Indices Chi-square; df p-value BBFI BBNFI CFI	22.15;12 0.035 1.000 1.000 1.000	6.940;12 0.861 1.000 1.000 1.000	12.40;12 .413 1.000 1.000 1.000

[a] = standardized coefficient, [b] = standard error, [c] = t-value

v1 = gnp, v2 = pricereg, v3 = mktfocus, v4 = r&dexpd, v5 = frginvst, v6 = innovat, v7 = gblsales

TABLE A.3. Global Innovation Model

Paths	Overall	Industrialized	Developing
v3,v1 Economic Env → Mkt/Ind Structure	-0.191[a] 0.190[b] -1.037[c]	-0.079 0.296 -0.226	-.186 .258 -.746
v3,v2 Regulation → Mkt/Ind Structure	-0.212 0.190 -1.147	0.137 0.296 0.461	-.313 .258 -1.258
v4,v1 Economic Env → Innovation Invst	0.182 0.158 1.085	0.500 0.158 2.759	.468 .235 2.118
v4,v2 Regulation → Innovation Invst	-0.490 0.159 -2.905	-0.632 0.159 -3.467	.115 .244 .501
v4,v3 Mkt/Ind Structure → Innovation Invst	-0.057 0.157 -0.334	0.209 0.160 1.143	-.230 .239 -.987
v5,v4 Innovation Invst → Foreign Mkt Invst	0.901 0.084 10.794	0.847 0.166 5.283	.890 .120 7.319
v6,v4 Innovation Invst → Global Innovation	1.562 0.170 9.313	1.539 0.234 6.889	-.885 .497 -1.672
v6,v5 Foreign Mkt Invst → Global Innovation	-0.776 0.168 -4.627	-0.885 0.226 -3.962	.947 .504 1.790
v7,v6 Global Innovation→ Global Sales	0.896 0.904 10.502	0.849 0.163 5.318	-.008 .267 -.031
Fit Indices Chi-square; df p-value BBFI BBNFI CFI	22.80;12 0.046 1.000 1.000 1.000	6.641;12 0.88 1.000 1.000 1.000	12.485;12 .407 0.995 1.000 1.000

[a] = standardized coefficient, [b] = standard error, [c] = t-value

v1 = gnp, v2 = pricereg, v3 = mktgrwth, v4 = r&dexpd, v5 = frginvst, v6 = innovat, v7 = gblsales

TABLE A.4. Global Innovation Model

Paths	Overall	Industrialized	Developing
v3,v1 Economic Env → Mkt/Ind Structure	-.421[a] .184[b] -2.408[c]	0.069 0.284 0.242	.036 .262 .135
v3,v2 Regulation → Mkt/Ind Structure	-.171 .184 -.978	-0.300 0.284 -1.047	-.164 .262 -.621
v4,v1 Economic Env → Innovation Invst	.114 .171 .628	0.499 0.157 2.763	.489 .182 2.863
v4,v2 Regulation → Innovation Invst	-.510 .158 -3.042	-0.671 0.164 -3.549	.278 .184 1.606
v4,v3 Mkt/Ind Structure → Innovation Invst	-.186 .165 -1.008	-0.225 0.166 -1.188	.553 .185 3.191
v5,v4 Innovation Invst → Foreign Mkt Invst	.901 .086 10.598	0.847 0.166 5.275	.890 .120 7.319
v6,v4 Innovation Invst → Global Innovation	1.562 .173 9.140	1.538 0.234 6.887	-.885 .497 -1.672
v6,v5 Foreign Mkt Invst→ Global Innovation	-.776 .172 -4.540	-0.885 0.226 -3.962	.947 .504 1.790
v7,v6 Global Innovation → Global Sales	.896 .088 10.310	0.848 0.164 5.314	-.008 .267 -.031
Fit Indices Chi-square; df p-value BBFI BBNFI CFI	33.73;12 0.001 1.000 1.000 1.000	8.76;12 0.72 1.000 1.000 1.000	13.62 .325 0.999 1.000 1.000

[a] = standardized coefficient, [b] = standard error, [c] = t-value

v1 = gnp, v2 = pricereg, v3 = mktconc, v4 = r&dexpd, v5 = frginvst, v6 = innovat, v7 = gblsales

TABLE A.5. Global Innovation Model

Paths	Overall	Industrialized	Developing
v3,v1 Economic Env → Mkt/Ind Structure	0.431[a] 0.174[b] 2.483[c]	0.578 0.241 2.382	-.029 .262 -.112
v3,v2 Regulation → Mkt/Ind Structure	-0.009 0.174 -0.051	0.130 0.241 0.534	-.175 .262 -.666
v4,v1 Economic Env → Innovation Invst	0.140 0.074 1.893	0.261 0.127 2.049	.576 .220 2.536
v4,v2 Regulation → Innovation Invst	-0.055 0.067 -0.820	-0.058 0.104 -0.558	-.329 .223 -1.595
v4,v3 Mkt/Ind Structure → Innovation Invst	0.868 0.074 11.774	0.768 0.129 5.975	-.262 .224 -1.267
v5,v4 Innovation Invst → Foreign Mkt Invst	0.913 0.079 11.599	0.877 0.145 6.043	.893 .118 7.416
v6,v4 Innovation Invst → Global Innovation	1.589 0.168 9.433	1.612 0.226 7.131	-.896 .496 -1.676
v6,v5 Foreign Mkt Invst → Global Innovation	-0.779 0.168 -4.627	-0.896 0.226 -3.962	.957 .504 1.790
v7,v6 Global Innovation→ Global Sales	0.906 0.082 11.089	0.868 0.150 5.807	-.008 .267 -.031
Fit Indices Chi-square; df p-value BBFI BBNFI CFI	32.41;12 0.001 1.000 1.000 1.000	13.76;12 0.315 1.000 1.000 1.000	11.622;12 .476 0.998 1.000 1.000

[a] = standardized coefficient, [b] = standard error, [c] = t-value

v1 = gnp, v2 = apptime, v3 = mktsize, v4 = r&dexpd, v5 = frginvst, v6 = innovat, v7 = gblsales

TABLE A.6. Global Innovation Model

Paths	Overall	Industrialized	Developing
v3,v1	-0.530[a]	-0.322	-.342
Economic Env →	0.163[b]	0.252	.250
Mkt/Ind Structure	-3.394[c]	-1.306	-1.363
v3,v2	0.247	0.476	-.035
Regulation →	0.163	0.252	.250
Mkt/Ind Structure	1.583	1.928	-.141
v4,v1	0.572	0.821	.404
Economic Env →	0.198	0.208	.225
Innovation Invst	2.927	3.938	1.942
v4,v2	-0.09	-0.130	-.294
Regulation →	0.173	0.224	.211
Innovation Invst	-0.523	-0.578	-1.502
v4,v3	0.110	0.359	-.353
Mkt/Ind Structure →	0.195	0.232	.226
Innovation Invst	0.547	1.516	-1.696
v5,v4	0.913	0.877	.893
Innovation Invst →	0.079	0.145	.118
Foreign Mkt Invst	11.602	6.043	7.416
v6,v4	1.589	1.612	-.896
Innovation Invst →	0.168	0.226	.496
Global Innovation	9.433	7.131	-1.676
v6,v5	-0.779	-0.896	.957
Foreign Mkt Invst →	0.168	0.226	.504
Global Innovation	-4.627	-3.962	1.790
v7,v6	0.906	0.868	-.008
Global Innovation →	0.082	0.150	.267
Global Sales	11.092	5.807	-.031
Fit Indices			
Chi-square, df	17.5;12	11.51;12	11.29;12
p-value	0.1303	0.485	.503
BBFI	1.000	1.000	0.998
BBNFI	1.000	1.000	1.000
CFI	1.000	1.000	1.000

[a] = standardized coefficient, [b] = standard error, [c] = t-value

v1 = gnp, v2 = apptime, v3 = mktfocus, v4 = r&dexpd, v5 = frginvst, v6 = innovat, v7 = gblsales

TABLE A.7. Global Innovation Model

Paths	Overall	Industrialized	Developing
v3,v1 Economic Env → Mkt/Ind Structure	-0.066[a] 0.192[b] -0.346[c]	-0.197 0.281 -0.706	.033 .267 .123
v3,v2 Regulation → Mkt/Ind Structure	0.058 0.192 0.300	0.329 0.281 1.180	-.054 .267 -.202
v4,v1 Economic Env → Innovation Invst	0.514 0.167 3.116	0.731 0.214 3.403	.532 .220 2.611
v4,v2 Regulation → Innovation Invst	-0.062 0.167 -0.378	-0.002 0.222 -0.009	-.297 .220 -1.455
v4,v3 Mkt/Ind Structure → Innovation Invst	0.001 0.167 0.008	0.131 0.225 0.577	-.253 .220 -1.241
v5,v4 Innovation Invst → Foreign Mkt Invst	0.913 0.079 11.603	0.877 0.145 6.043	.893 .118 7.416
v6,v4 Innovation Invst → Global Innovation	1.589 0.168 9.433	1.613 0.226 7.131	-.896 .496 -1.676
v6,v5 Foreign Mkt Invst → Global Innovation	-0.779 0.168 -4.627	-0.896 0.226 -3.962	.957 .504 1.790
v7,v6 Global Innovation → Global Sales	0.906 0.082 11.092	0.868 0.150 5.807	-.008 .267 -.031
Fit Indices Chi-square; df p-value BBFI BBNFI CFI	48.79;12 0.001 1.000 1.000 1.000	7.726;12 0.8061 1.000 1.000 1.000	10.357;12 .584 0.996 1.000 1.000

[a] = standardized coefficient, [b] = standard error, [c] = t-value

v1 = gnp, v2 = apptime, v3 = mktgrwth, v4 = r&dexpd, v5 = frginvst, v6 = innovat, v7 = gblsales

TABLE A.8. Global Innovation Model

Paths	Overall	Industrialized	Developing
v3,v1 Economic Env → Mkt/Ind Structure	-0.362[a] 0.180[b] -2.05[c]	0.225 0.293 0.768	.086 .263 .327
v3,v2 Regulation → Mkt/Ind Structure	0.166 0.180 0.938	0.033 0.293 0.113	.113 .263 .429
v4,v1 Economic Env → Innovation Invst	0.474 0.178 2.699	0.722 0.217 3.311	.478 .172 3.003
v4,v2 Regulation → Innovation Invst	-0.044 0.168 -0.264	0.044 0.212 0.205	-.342 .172 -2.143
v4,v3 Mkt/Ind Structure → Innovation Invst	-0.111 0.177 -0.621	-0.071 0.217 -0.326	.548 .174 3.420
v5,v4 Innovation Invst → Foreign Mkt Invst	0.913 0.079 11.604	0.877 0.145 6.043	.893 .118 7.416
v6,v4 Innovation Invst → Global Innovation	1.58 0.168 9.433	1.613 0.226 7.131	-.896 .496 -1.676
v6,v5 Foreign Mkt Invst → Global Innovation	-0.779 0.168 -4.627	-0.896 0.226 -3.962	.957 .504 1.790
v7,v6 Global Innovation→ Global Sales	0.906 0.082 11.093	0.868 0.150 5.807	-.008 .267 -.031
Fit Indices Chi-square; df p-value BBFI BBNFI CFI	41.26;12 0.001 1.000 1.000 1.000	10.631;12 0.560 1.000 1.000 1.000	13.007;12 .368 .999 1.000 1.000

[a] = standardized coefficient, [b] = standard error, [c] = t-value

v1 = gnp, v2 = apptime, v3 = mktconc, v4 = r&dexpd, v5 = frginvst, v6 = innovat, v7 = gblsales

TABLE A.9. Global Innovation Model

Paths	Overall	Industrialized	Developing
v3,v1 Economic Env → Mkt/Ind Structure	0.372[a] 0.153[b] 2.726[c]	0.984 0.054 18.48	.618 .221 3.263
v3,v2 Regulation → Mkt/Ind Structure	-0.60 0.153 -4.406	0.034 0.054 0.630	-.340 .221 -1.792
v4,v1 Economic Env → Innovation Invst	0.048 0.073 0.744	0.613 0.479 1.095	-.032 .337 -.096
v4,v2 Regulation → Innovation Invst	-0.184 0.084 -2.481	-0.359 0.086 -3.564	-.105 .282 -.371
v4,v3 Mkt/Ind Structure → Innovation Invst	0.817 0.081 10.207	0.267 0.469 0.476	-.300 .308 -.835
v5,v4 Innovation Invst → Foreign Mkt Invst	0.929 0.070 13.031	0.842 0.169 5.186	.878 .128 6.867
v6,v4 Innovation Invst → Global Innovation	1.62 0.165 9.600	1.528 0.236 6.853	-.830 .504 -1.649
v6,v5 Foreign Mkt Invst → Global Innovation	-0.785 0.168 -4.627	-0.884 0.226 -3.962	.901 .504 1.790
v7,v6 Global Innovation→ Global Sales	0.920 0.074 12.157	0.846 0.165 5.258	-.008 .267 -.031
Fit Indices Chi-square; df p-value BBFI BBNFI CFI	27.29;12 0.007 1.000 1.000 1.000	9.499;12 0.659 1.000 1.000 1.000	11.604;12 .477 1.000 1.000 1.000

[a] = standardized coefficient, [b] = standard error, [c] = t-value

v1 = pop, v2 = pricereg, v3 = mktsize, v4 = r&dexpd, v5 = frginvst, v6 = innovat, v7 = gblsales

TABLE A.10. Global Innovation Model

Paths	Overall	Industrialized	Developing
v3,v1	0.155[a]	0.503	.317
Economic Env →	0.171[b]	0.250	.244
Mkt/Ind Structure	0.880[c]	2.459	1.265
v3,v2	0.376	0.534	.139
Regulation →	0.171	0.250	.244
Mkt/Ind Structure	2.137	2.609	.554
v4,v1	0.346	0.876	-.073
Economic Env →	0.144	0.106	.247
Innovation Invst	2.736	7.013	-.295
v4,v2	-0.689	-.350	.060
Regulation →	0.153	.109	.237
Innovation Invst	-5.112	-2.746	.251
v4,v3	0.039	-.000	-.454
Mkt/Ind Structure →	0.159	.103	.257
Innovation Invst	0.285	-.002	-1.817
v5,v4	0.929	.842	.878
Innovation Invst →	0.070	.170	.128
Foreign Mkt Invst	13.03	5.168	6.867
v6,v4	1.62	1.526	-.830
Innovation Invst →	0.165	.236	.504
Global Innovation	9.60	6.846	-1.649
v6,v5	-0.785	-.883	.901
Foreign Mkt Invst →	0.168	.226	.504
Global Innovation	-4.627	-3.962	1.790
v7,v6	0.920	.845	-.008
Global Innovation →	0.074	0.166	.267
Global Sales	12.159	5.247	-.031
Fit Indices			
Chi-square; df	19.83;12	8.23;12	13.09;12
p-value	0.070	0.766	.362
BBFI	1.000	1.000	1.000
BBNFI	1.000	1.000	1.000
CFI	1.000	1.000	1.000

[a] = standardized coefficient, [b] = standard error, [c] = t-value

v1 = pop, v2 = pricereg, v3 = mktfocus, v4 = r&dexpd, v5 = frginvst, v6 = innovat, v7 = gblsales

TABLE A.11. Global Innovation Model

Paths	Overall	Industrialized	Developing
v3,v1 Economic Env → Mkt/Ind Structure	0.093[a] 0.191[b] .489[c]	.089 .296 .306	.25 .256 1.036
v3,v2 Regulation → Mkt/Ind Structure	−.120 .191 −.630	.231 .296 .793	−.347 .256 −1.434
v4,v1 Economic Env → Innovation Invst	.358 .141 2.882	.863 .079 9.365	−.146 .260 −.559
v4,v2 Regulation → Innovation Invst	−.686 .142 −5.507	−.383 .080 −4.054	−.104 .269 −.388
v4,v3 Mkt/Ind Structure → Innovation Invst	−.088 .141 −.700	.138 .080 1.454	−.290 .262 −1.043
v5,v4 Innovation Invst → Foreign Mkt Invst	.929 .070 13.040	.842 .170 5.172	.878 .128 6.867
v6,v4 Innovation Invst → Global Innovation	1.629 0.165 9.601	1.527 .236 6.848	−.830 .504 −1.649
v6,v5 Foreign Mkt Invst → Global Innovation	−.785 0.168 −4.627	−.883 .226 −3.962	.901 .504 1.790
v7,v6 Global Innovation → Global Sales	.920 .074 12.163	.845 .166 5.249	−.008 .267 −.031
Fit Indices Chi-square; df p-value BBFI BBNFI CFI	20.81;12 0.053 1.000 1.000 1.000	7.932;12 .790 1.000 1.000 1.000	12.29;12 .422 1.000 1.000 1.000

[a] = standardized coefficient, [b] = standard error, [c] = t-value

v1 = pop, v2 = pricereg, v3 = mktgrwth, v4 = r&dexpd, v5 = frginvst, v6 = innovat,
v7 = gblsales

TABLE A.12. Global Innovation Model

Paths	Overall	Industrialized	Developing
v3,v1 Economic Env → Mkt/Ind Structure	0.029[a] 0.194[b] .149[c]	-.304 .273 -1.227	.092 .262 .356
v3,v2 Regulation → Mkt/Ind Structure	.117 .194 .601	-.484 .273 -1.957	-.243 .262 -.944
v4,v1 Economic Env → Innovation Invst	.356 .139 2.907	.876 .091 8.208	-.280 .205 -1.366
v4,v2 Regulation → Innovation Invst	-.655 .140 -5.307	-.349 .099 -3.001	.148 .210 .703
v4,v3 Mkt/Ind Structure → Innovation Invst	-.174 .141 -1.409	.001 .094 .011	.628 .208 2.970
v5,v4 Innovation Invst → Foreign Mkt Invst	.929 .071 12.799	.842 .170 5.172	.878 .128 6.867
v6,v4 Innovation Invst → Global Innovation	1.629 .168 9.420	1.527 .236 6.849	-.830 .504 -1.649
v6,v5 Foreign Mkt Invst→ Global Innovation	-.785 .172 -4.540	-.884 .226 -3.962	.901 .504 1.790
v7,v6 Global Innovation → Global Sales	.920 .076 11.936	.846 .165 5.252	-.008 .267 -.031
Fit Indices Chi-square; df p-value BBFI BBNFI CFI	25.44;12 0.012 1.000 1.000 1.000	8.476;12 .746 1.000 1.000 1.000	13.59;12 .327 1.000 1.000 1.000

[a] = standardized coefficient, [b] = standard error, [c] = t-value

v1 = pop, v2 = pricereg, v3 = mktconc, v4 = r&dexpd, v5 = frginvst, v6 = innovat, v7 = gblsales

TABLE A.13. Global Innovation Model

Paths	Overall	Industrialized	Developing
v3,v1 Economic Env → Mkt/Ind Structure	0.127[a] 0.189[b] .676[c]	.983 .055 17.934	.457 .235 1.928
v3,v2 Regulation → Mkt/Ind Structure	.158 .189 .839	.024 .055 .434	-.070 .235 -.297
v4,v1 Economic Env → Innovation Invst	-.074 .070 -1.05	.888 .609 1.469	-.142 .285 -.501
v4,v2 Regulation → Innovation Invst	-.031 .071 -.446	-.040 .112 -.365	-.118 .254 -.468
v4,v3 Mkt/Ind Structure → Innovation Invst	.943 .071 13.24	.043 .612 .071	-.232 .288 -.816
v5,v4 Innovation Invst → Foreign Mkt Invst	.911 .079 11.49	.879 .144 6.106	.880 .127 6.920
v6,v4 Innovation Invst → Global Innovation	1.58 .168 9.41	1.618 .226 7.148	-.837 .503 -1.652
v6,v5 Foreign Mkt Invst → Global Innovation	-.779 .168 -4.62	-.897 .226 -3.962	.907 .504 1.790
v7,v6 Global Innovation → Global Sales	.904 .082 11.009	.870 .149 5.849	-.008 .267 -.031
Fit Indices Chi-square; df p-value BBFI BBNFI CFI	27.9;12 0.005 1.000 1.000 1.000	9.691;12 .643 1.000 1.000 1.000	9.972;12 .618 1.000 1.000 1.000

[a] = standardized coefficient, [b] = standard error, [c] = t-value

v1 = pop, v2 = apptime, v3 = mktsize, v4 = r&dexpd, v5 = frginvst, v6 = innovat, v7 = gblsales

TABLE A.14. Global Innovation Model

Paths	Overall	Industrialized	Developing
v3,v1 Economic Env → Mkt/Ind Structure	0.348[a] 0.180[b] 1.951[c]	.138 .267 .511	.369 .245 1.496
v3,v2 Regulation → Mkt/Ind Structure	.144 .180 .807	.423 .267 1.569	-.099 .245 -.399
v4,v1 Economic Env → Innovation Invst	.136 .199 .686	.949 .106 9.021	-.075 .249 -.301
v4,v2 Regulation → Innovation Invst	.153 .189 .809	.017 .116 .148	-.148 .233 -.639
v4,v3 Mkt/Ind Structure → Innovation Invst	-.229 .199 -1.14	-.133 .118 -1.149	-.468 .253 -1.880
v5,v4 Innovation Invst → Foreign Mkt Invst	.911 .079 11.493	.879 .144 6.106	.880 .127 6.920
v6,v4 Innovation Invst → Global Innovation	1.58 .168 9.418	1.618 .226 7.148	-.837 .503 -1.652
v6,v5 Foreign Mkt Invst → Global Innovation	-.779 .168 -4.627	-.897 .226 -3.962	.907 .504 1.790
v7,v6 Global Innovation → Global Sales	.904 .082 11.012	.870 .149 5.849	-.008 .267 -.031
Fit Indices Chi-square; df p-value BBFI BBNFI CFI	15.92;12 0.19 1.000 1.000 1.000	7.790;12 .780 1.000 1.000 1.000	11.96;12 .448 1.000 1.000 1.000

[a] = standardized coefficient, [b] = standard error, [c] = t-value

v1 = pop, v2 = apptime, v3 = mktfocus, v4 = r&dexpd, v5 = frginvst, v6 = innovat, v7 = gblsales

TABLE A.15. Global Innovation Model

Paths	Overall	Industrialized	Developing
v3,v1 Economic Env → Mkt/Ind Structure	0.046[a] 0.192[b] .237[c]	-.115 .285 -.406	.024 .267 .091
v3,v2 Regulation → Mkt/Ind Structure	.045 .192 .234	.325 .285 1.148	-.033 .267 -.123
v4,v1 Economic Env → Innovation Invst	.058 .191 .305	.941 .109 8.723	-.241 .250 -.971
v4,v2 Regulation → Innovation Invst	.121 .191 .634	-.069 .114 -.606	-.110 .250 -.443
v4,v3 Mkt/Ind Structure → Innovation Invst	-.032 .191 -.168	.090 .114 .786	-.252 .250 -1.015
v5,v4 Innovation Invst → Foreign Mkt Invst	.911 .079 11.49	.879 .144 6.106	.880 .127 6.920
v6,v4 Innovation Invst → Global Innovation	1.58 .168 9.41	1.618 .226 7.148	-.837 .503 -1.652
v6,v5 Foreign Mkt Invst → Global Innovation	-.779 .168 -4.62	-.897 .226 -3.962	.907 .504 1.790
v7,v6 Global Innovation → Global Sales	.904 .082 11.01	.870 .149 5.849	-.008 .267 -.031
Fit Indices Chi-square; df p-value BBFI BBNFI CFI	15.66;12 0.20 1.000 1.000 1.000	8.064;12 .780 1.000 1.000 1.000	10.876;12 .539 1.000 1.000 1.000

[a] = standardized coefficient, [b] = standard error, [c] = t-value

v1 = pop, v2 = apptime, v3 = mktgrwth, v4 = r&dexpd, v5 = frginvst, v6 = innovat, v7 = gblsales

TABLE A.16. Global Innovation Model

Paths	Overall	Industrialized	Developing
v3,v1 Economic Env → Mkt/Ind Structure	0.095[a] 0.191[b] .498[c]	-.017 .301 -.057	-.021 .264 -.078
v3,v2 Regulation → Mkt/Ind Structure	.066 .191 .347	.065 .301 .215	.148 .264 .560
v4,v1 Economic Env → Innovation Invst	.083 .184 .450	.932 .106 8.838	-.235 .200 -1.179
v4,v2 Regulation → Innovation Invst	.138 .184 .750	-.046 .106 -.437	-.193 .203 -.961
v4,v3 Mkt/Ind Structure → Innovation Invst	-.275 .185 -1.49	.104 .106 .984	.618 .203 3.072
v5,v4 Innovation Invst → Foreign Mkt Invst	.911 .079 11.49	.879 .144 6.106	.880 .127 6.920
v6,v4 Innovation Invst → Global Innovation	1.58 .168 9.41	1.618 .226 7.148	-.837 .503 -1.652
v6,v5 Foreign Mkt Invst → Global Innovation	-.779 .168 -4.62	-.897 .226 -3.962	.907 .504 1.790
v7,v6 Global Innovation → Global Sales	.904 .082 11.01	.870 .149 5.849	-.008 .267 -.031
Fit Indices Chi-square; df p-value BBFI BBNFI CFI	16.43;12 0.17 1.000 1.000 1.000	8.804;12 .719 1.000 1.000 1.000	13.483;12 .334 1.000 1.000 1.000

[a] = standardized coefficient, [b] = standard error, [c] = t-value

v1 = pop, v2 = apptime, v3 = mktconc, v4 = r&dexpd, v5 = frginvst, v6 = innovat, v7 = gblsales

TABLE A.17. Global Innovation Model

Paths	Overall	Industrialized	Developing
v3,v1 Economic Env → Mkt/Ind Structure	0.190[a] 0.167[b] 1.084[c]	.423 .225 1.725	-.129 .265 -.486
v3,v2 Regulation → Mkt/Ind Structure	-.365 .167 -2.078	-.397 .225 -1.618	-.030 .265 -.113
v4,v1 Economic Env → Innovation Invst	.026 .066 .374	.192 .090 1.850	.483 .233 2.208
v4,v2 Regulation → Innovation Invst	-.165 .070 -2.218	-.330 .089 -3.217	.180 .231 .832
v4,v3 Mkt/Ind Structure → Innovation Invst	.856 .075 11.30	.685 .107 6.049	-.218 .232 -.995
v5,v4 Innovation Invst → Foreign Mkt Invst	.135 .203 .710	-.241 .334 -.825	.580 .209 2.665
v6,v4 Innovation Invst → Global Innovation	.876 .098 9.101	.691 .155 4.677	-.220 .298 -.694
v6,v5 Foreign Mkt Invst → Global Innovation	-.105 .092 -1.089	-.402 .136 -2.720	.308 .311 .972
v7,v6 Global Innovation → Global Sales	.896 .086 10.489	.848 .164 5.306	-.008 .267 -.031
Fit Indices Chi-square; df p-value BBFI BBNFI CFI	24.99;12 0.014 1.000 1.000 1.000	9.8;12 .633 1.000 1.000 1.000	13.889;12 .307 1.000 1.000 1.000

[a] = standardized coefficient, [b] = standard error, [c] = t-value

v1 = gnp, v2 = pricereg, v3 = mktsize, v4 = r&dexpd, v5 = frgcomm, v6 = innovat, v7 = gblsales

TABLE A.18. Global Innovation Model

Paths	Overall	Industrialized	Developing
v3,v1 Economic Env → Mkt/Ind Structure	-.336[a] 0.168[b] -1.911[c]	-.164 .287 -.562	-.256 .247 -1.008
v3,v2 Regulation → Mkt/Ind Structure	.226 .168 1.287	.191 .287 .655	.181 .247 .714
v4,v1 Economic Env → Innovation Invst	.241 .163 1.385	.552 .130 3.695	.417 .224 1.980
v4,v2 Regulation → Innovation Invst	-.511 .158 -3.044	-.684 .131 -4.554	.252 .221 1.217
v4,v3 Mkt/Ind Structure → Innovation Invst	.147 .176 .825	.416 .135 2.732	-.372 .234 -1.735
v5,v4 Innovation Invst → Foreign Mkt Invst	.136 .203 .711	-.242 .332 -.829	.580 .209 2.665
v6,v4 Innovation Invst → Global Innovation	.877 .098 9.111	.693 .155 4.699	-.220 .298 -.694
v6,v5 Foreign Mkt Invst → Global Innovation	-.105 .092 -1.089	-.401 .136 -2.720	.308 .311 .972
v7,v6 Global Innovation → Global Sales	.896 .086 10.498	.849 .163 5.323	-.008 .267 -.031
Fit Indices Chi-square; df p-value BBFI BBNFI CFI	22.35;12 0.033 1.000 1.000 1.000	7.819;12 .799 1.000 1.000 1.000	11.934;12 .450 1.000 1.000 1.000

[a] = standardized coefficient, [b] = standard error, [c] = t-value

v1 = gnp, v2 = pricereg, v3 = mktfocus, v4 = r&dexpd, v5 = frgcomm, v6 = innovat, v7 = gblsales

TABLE A.19. Global Innovation Model

Paths	Overall	Industrialized	Developing
v3,v1 Economic Env → Mkt/Ind Structure	-0.191[a] 0.190[b] -1.037[c]	-.079 .296 -.266	-.186 .258 -.746
v3,v2 Regulation → Mkt/Ind Structure	-.212 .190 -1.147	.137 .296 .461	-.313 .258 -1.258
v4,v1 Economic Env → Innovation Invst	.182 .158 1.085	.500 .158 2.759	.468 .235 2.118
v4,v2 Regulation → Innovation Invst	-.490 .159 -2.905	-.632 .159 -3.467	.115 .244 .501
v4,v3 Mkt/Ind Structure → Innovation Invst	-.057 .157 -.334	.209 .160 1.143	-.230 .239 -.987
v5,v4 Innovation Invst → Foreign Mkt Invst	.136 .203 .711	-.242 .333 -.828	.580 .209 2.665
v6,v4 Innovation Invst → Global Innovation	.877 .098 9.115	.692 .155 4.693	-.220 .298 -.694
v6,v5 Foreign Mkt Invst → Global Innovation	-.105 .092 -1.089	-.401 .136 -2.720	.308 .311 .972
v7,v6 Global Innovation → Global Sales	.896 .086 10.502	.849 .163 5.318	-.008 .267 -.031
Fit Indices Chi-square; df p-value BBFI BBNFI CFI	20.87;12 0.05 1.000 1.000 1.000	7.267;12 .839 1.000 1.000 1.000	13.028;12 .366 0.980 0.997 0.998

[a] = standardized coefficient, [b] = standard error, [c] = t-value

v1 = gnp, v2 = pricereg, v3 = mktgrwth, v4 = r&dexpd, v5 = frgcomm, v6 = innovat, v7 = gblsales

TABLE A.20. Global Innovation Model

Paths	Overall	Industrialized	Developing
v3,v1 Economic Env → Mkt/Ind Structure	-.421[a] 0.181[b] -2.454[c]	.069 .284 .242	.036 .262 .135
v3,v2 Regulation → Mkt/Ind Structure	-.171 .181 -.996	-.300 .284 -1.047	-.164 .262 -.621
v4,v1 Economic Env → Innovation Invst	.114 .168 .640	.499 .157 2.763	.489 .182 2.863
v4,v2 Regulation → Innovation Invst	-.510 .155 -3.100	-.671 .164 -3.549	.278 .184 1.606
v4,v3 Mkt/Ind Structure → Innovation Invst	-.186 .162 -1.027	-.225 .166 -1.188	.553 .185 3.191
v5,v4 Innovation Invst → Foreign Mkt Invst	.136 .202 .711	-.242 .333 -.827	.580 .209 2.665
v6,v4 Innovation Invst → Global Innovation	.877 .098 9.12	.692 .155 4.687	-.220 .298 -.694
v6,v5 Foreign Mkt Invst → Global Innovation	-.105 .092 -1.089	-.401 .136 -2.720	.308 .311 .972
v7,v6 Global Innovation → Global Sales	.896 .086 10.506	.848 .164 5.314	-.008 .267 -.031
Fit Indices Chi-square; df p-value BBFI BBNFI CFI	20.83;12 0.05 1.000 1.000 1.000	11.399;12 .49 1.000 1.000 1.000	14.227;12 .286 0.991 0.998 0.999

[a] = standardized coefficient, [b] = standard error, [c] = t-value

v1 = gnp, v2 = pricereg, v3 = mktconc, v4 = r&dexpd, v5 = frgcomm, v6 = innovat, v7 = gblsales

TABLE A.21. Global Innovation Model

Paths	Overall	Industrialized	Developing
v3,v1 Economic Env → Mkt/Ind Structure	0.432[a] 0.174[b] 2.486[c]	.578 .241 2.382	-.029 .262 -.112
v3,v2 Regulation → Mkt/Ind Structure	-.009 .174 -.051	.130 .241 .534	-.175 .262 -.666
v4,v1 Economic Env → Innovation Invst	.140 .074 1.901	.261 .127 2.048	.576 .220 2.536
v4,v2 Regulation → Innovation Invst	-.053 .067 -.799	-.058 .104 -.557	-.329 .223 -1.595
v4,v3 Mkt/Ind Structure → Innovation Invst	.867 .074 11.773	.768 .129 5.975	-.262 .224 -1.267
v5,v4 Innovation Invst → Foreign Mkt Invst	.146 .188 .764	-.275 .291 -.947	.585 .206 2.700
v6,v4 Innovation Invst → Global Innovation	.892 .091 9.785	.725 .136 5.321	-.223 .295 -.700
v6,v5 Foreign Mkt Invst → Global Innovation	-.099 .092 -1.089	-.371 .136 -2.720	.310 .311 .972
v7,v6 Global Innovation → Global Sales	.906 .082 11.094	.868 .150 5.807	-.008 .267 -.031
Fit Indices Chi-square; df p-value BBFI BBNFI CFI	22.10;12 0.036 1.000 1.000 1.000	10.005;12 .615 1.000 1.000 1.000	10.647;12 .559 0.990 1.000 1.000

[a] = standardized coefficient, [b] = standard error, [c] = t-value

v1 = gnp, v2 = apptime, v3 = mktsize, v4 = r&dexpd, v5 = frgcomm, v6 = innovat, v7 = gblsales

TABLE A.22. Global Innovation Model

Paths	Overall	Industrialized	Developing
v3,v1 Economic Env → Mkt/Ind Structure	-.529[a] .163[b] -3.38[c]	-.322 .252 -1.306	-.342 .250 -1.363
v3,v2 Regulation → Mkt/Ind Structure	.247 .163 1.58	.476 .252 1.928	-.035 .250 -.141
v4,v1 Economic Env → Innovation Invst	.573 .195 2.932	.821 .208 3.938	.404 .225 1.942
v4,v2 Regulation → Innovation Invst	-.09 .173 -.526	-.130 .224 -.578	-.294 .211 -1.502
v4,v3 Mkt/Ind Structure → Innovation Invst	.110 .195 .547	.359 .232 1.516	-.353 .226 -1.696
v5,v4 Innovation Invst → Foreign Mkt Invst	.146 .188 .765	-.275 .291 -.947	.585 .206 2.700
v6,v4 Innovation Invst → Global Innovation	.892 .091 9.786	.725 .136 5.321	-.223 .295 -.700
v6,v5 Foreign Mkt Invst → Global Innovation	-.099 .092 -1.089	-.371 .136 -2.720	.310 .311 .972
v7,v6 Global Innovation → Global Sales	.906 .082 11.094	.868 .150 5.807	-.008 .267 -.031
Fit Indices Chi-square; df p-value BBFI BBNFI CFI	19.11;12 0.08 1.000 1.000 1.000	9.440;12 .664 1.000 1.000 1.000	11.309;12 .502 0.983 1.000 1.000

[a] = standardized coefficient, [b] = standard error, [c] = t-value

v1 = gnp, v2 = apptime, v3 = mktfocus, v4 = r&dexpd, v5 = frgcomm, v6 = innovat, v7 = gblsales

TABLE A.23. Global Innovation Model

Paths	Overall	Industrialized	Developing
v3,v1 Economic Env → Mkt/Ind Structure	-.065[a] .192[b] -.339[c]	-.197 .281 -.706	.033 .267 .123
v3,v2 Regulation → Mkt/Ind Structure	.058 .192 .301	.329 .281 1.180	-.054 .267 -.202
v4,v1 Economic Env → Innovation Invst	.515 .167 3.119	.731 .214 3.403	.532 .220 2.611
v4,v2 Regulation → Innovation Invst	-.063 .167 -.382	-.002 .222 -.009	-.297 .220 -1.455
v4,v3 Mkt/Ind Structure → Innovation Invst	.001 .167 .008	.131 .225 .577	-.253 .220 -1.241
v5,v4 Innovation Invst → Foreign Mkt Invst	.146 .188 .765	-.275 .291 -.947	.585 .206 2.700
v6,v4 Innovation Invst → Global Innovation	.892 .091 9.786	.725 .136 5.321	-.223 .295 -.700
v6,v5 Foreign Mkt Invst → Global Innovation	-.099 .092 -1.089	-.371 .136 -2.720	.310 .311 .972
v7,v6 Global Innovation → Global Sales	.906 .082 11.094	.868 .150 5.808	-.008 .267 -.031
Fit Indices Chi-square; df p-value BBFI BBNFI CFI	16.82;12 0.156 1.000 1.000 1.000	9.373;12 .67 1.000 1.000 1.000	9.937;12 .62 0.990 1.000 1.000

[a] = standardized coefficient, [b] = standard error, [c] = t-value

v1 = gnp, v2 = apptime, v3 = mktgrwth, v4 = r&dexpd, v5 = frgcomm, v6 = innovat, v7 = gblsales

TABLE A.24. Global Innovation Model

Paths	Overall	Industrialized	Developing
v3,v1 Economic Env → Mkt/Ind Structure	-.361[a] .180[b] -2.041[c]	.225 .293 .768	.086 .263 .327
v3,v2 Regulation → Mkt/Ind Structure	.166 .180 .938	.033 .293 .113	.113 .263 .429
v4,v1 Economic Env → Innovation Invst	.475 .178 2.703	.722 .217 3.311	.478 .172 3.003
v4,v2 Regulation → Innovation Invst	-.045 .168 -.273	.044 .212 .205	-.342 .172 -2.143
v4,v3 Mkt/Ind Structure → Innovation Invst	-.110 .177 -.621	-.071 .217 -.326	.548 .174 3.420
v5,v4 Innovation Invst → Foreign Mkt Invst	.146 .188 .765	-.275 .291 -.947	.585 .206 2.700
v6,v4 Innovation Invst → Global Innovation	.892 .091 9.786	.725 .136 5.321	-.223 .295 -.700
v6,v5 Foreign Mkt Invst → Global Innovation	-.099 .092 -1.089	-.371 .136 -2.720	.310 .311 .972
v7,v6 Global Innovation → Global Sales	.906 .081 11.095	.868 .150 5.807	-.008 .267 -.031
Fit Indices Chi-square; df p-value BBFI BBNFI CFI	41.93;12 0.001 1.000 1.000 1.000	11.771;12 .464 1.000 1.000 1.000	13.316;12 .346 1.000 1.000 1.000

[a] = standardized coefficient, [b] = standard error, [c] = t-value

v1 = gnp, v2 = apptime, v3 = mktconc, v4 = r&dexpd, v5 = frgcomm, v6 = innovat, v7 = gblsales

TABLE A.25. Global Innovation Model

Paths	Overall	Industrialized	Developing
v3,v1 Economic Env → Mkt/Ind Structure	0.371[a] 0.153[b] 2.72[c]	.984 .054 18.48	.618 .221 3.263
v3,v2 Regulation → Mkt/Ind Structure	-.601 .153 -4.412	.034 .054 .630	-.340 .221 -1.792
v4,v1 Economic Env → Innovation Invst	.046 .073 .714	.613 .479 1.095	-.032 .337 -.096
v4,v2 Regulation → Innovation Invst	-.186 .084 -2.507	-.359 .086 -3.564	-.105 .282 -.371
v4,v3 Mkt/Ind Structure → Innovation Invst	.816 .081 10.20	.267 .469 .476	-.300 .308 -.835
v5,v4 Innovation Invst → Foreign Mkt Invst	.163 .168 .859	-.238 .339 -.813	.556 .222 2.500
v6,v4 Innovation Invst → Global Innovation	.914 .081 10.966	.687 .157 4.613	-.207 .311 -.665
v6,v5 Foreign Mkt Invst → Global Innovation	-.091 .092 -1.089	-.405 .136 -2.720	.302 .311 .972
v7,v6 Global Innovation → Global Sales	.920 .074 12.165	.846 .165 5.258	-.008 .267 -.031
Fit Indices Chi-square; df p-value BBFI BBNFI CFI	21.24;12 0.046 1.000 1.000 1.000	11.216;12 .51 1.000 1.000 1.000	12.237;12 .426 0.992 1.000 1.000

[a] = standardized coefficient, [b] = standard error, [c] = t-value

v1 = pop, v2 = pricereg, v3 = mktsize, v4 = r&dexpd, v5 = frgcomm, v6 = innovat, v7 = gblsales

TABLE A.26. Global Innovation Model

Paths	Overall	Industrialized	Developing
v3,v1 Economic Env → Mkt/Ind Structure	0.155[a] 0.171[b] .880[c]	.503 .250 2.459	.317 .244 1.265
v3,v2 Regulation → Mkt/Ind Structure	.376 .171 2.137	.534 .250 2.609	.139 .244 .554
v4,v1 Economic Env → Innovation Invst	.346 .144 2.736	.876 .106 7.013	-.073 .247 -.295
v4,v2 Regulation → Innovation Invst	-.689 .153 -5.112	-.350 .109 -2.746	.060 .237 .251
v4,v3 Mkt/Ind Structure → Innovation Invst	.039 .159 .285	-.000 .103 -.002	-.454 .257 -1.817
v5,v4 Innovation Invst → Foreign Mkt Invst	.163 .168 .859	-.237 .340 -.810	.556 .222 2.500
v6,v4 Innovation Invst → Global Innovation	.914 .081 10.961	.687 .158 4.597	-.207 .311 -.665
v6,v5 Foreign Mkt Invst → Global Innovation	-.091 .092 -1.089	-.406 .136 -2.720	.302 .311 .972
v7,v6 Global Innovation → Global Sales	.920 .074 12.161	.845 .166 5.247	-.008 .267 -.031
Fit Indices Chi-square; df p-value BBFI BBNFI CFI	25.61;12 0.012 1.000 1.000 1.000	8.982;12 .704 1.000 1.000 1.000	13.709;12 .319 0.990 0.998 0.999

[a] = standardized coefficient, [b] = standard error, [c] = t-value

v1 = pop, v2 = pricereg, v3 = mktfocus, v4 = r&dexpd, v5 = frgcomm, v6 = innovat, v7 = gblsales

TABLE A.27. Global Innovation Model

Paths	Overall	Industrialized	Developing
v3,v1 Economic Env → Mkt/Ind Structure	0.095[a] 0.191[b] .501[c]	.089 .296 .306	.250 .256 1.036
v3,v2 Regulation → Mkt/Ind Structure	-.119 .191 -.625	.231 .296 .793	-.347 .256 -1.434
v4,v1 Economic Env → Innovation Invst	.360 .141 2.893	.863 .079 9.365	-.146 .260 -.559
v4,v2 Regulation → Innovation Invst	-.686 .142 -5.502	-.383 .080 -4.054	-.104 .269 -.388
v4,v3 Mkt/Ind Structure → Innovation Invst	-.088 .141 -.700	.138 .080 1.454	-.290 .262 -1.043
v5,v4 Innovation Invst → Foreign Mkt Invst	.163 .168 .859	-.237 .340 -.811	.556 .222 2.500
v6,v4 Innovation Invst → Global Innovation	.914 .081 10.963	.687 .158 4.601	-.207 .311 -.665
v6,v5 Foreign Mkt Invst → Global Innovation	-.091 .092 -1.089	-.406 .136 -2.720	.302 .311 .972
v7,v6 Global Innovation → Global Sales	.920 .074 12.163	.845 .166 5.249	-.008 .267 -.031
Fit Indices Chi-square; df p-value BBFI BBNFI CFI	21.06;12 0.049 1.000 1.000 1.000	8.792;12 .720 1.000 1.000 1.000	13.33;12 .345 1.000 1.000 1.000

[a] = standardized coefficient, [b] = standard error, [c] = t-value

v1 = pop, v2 = pricereg, v3 = mktgrwth, v4 = r&dexpd, v5 = frgcomm, v6 = innovat, v7 = gblsales

TABLE A.28. Global Innovation Model

Paths	Overall	Industrialized	Developing
v3,v1 Economic Env → Mkt/Ind Structure	0.029[a] 0.191[b] .152[c]	-.304 .273 -1.227	.092 .262 .356
v3,v2 Regulation → Mkt/Ind Structure	.117 .191 .612	-.484 .273 -1.957	-.243 .262 -.944
v4,v1 Economic Env → Innovation Invst	.356 .137 2.962	.876 .091 8.208	-.280 .205 -1.366
v4,v2 Regulation → Innovation Invst	-.655 .138 -5.408	-.349 .099 -3.001	.148 .210 .703
v4,v3 Mkt/Ind Structure → Innovation Invst	-.174 .138 -1.436	.001 .094 .011	.628 .208 2.970
v5,v4 Innovation Invst → Foreign Mkt Invst	.163 .168 .859	-.238 .340 -.811	.556 .222 2.500
v6,v4 Innovation Invst → Global Innovation	.914 .081 10.967	.687 .158 4.604	-.207 .311 -.665
v6,v5 Foreign Mkt Invst → Global Innovation	-.091 .092 -1.089	-.406 .136 -2.720	.302 .311 .972
v7,v6 Global Innovation → Global Sales	.920 .074 12.167	.846 .165 5.252	-.008 .267 -.031
Fit Indices Chi-square; df p-value BBFI BBNFI CFI	20.95;12 0.05 1.000 1.000 1.000	10.551;12 .567 1.000 1.000 1.000	14.020;12 .299 0.994 0.998 0.999

[a] = standardized coefficient, [b] = standard error, [c] = t-value

v1 = pop, v2 = pricereg, v3 = mktconc, v4 = r&dexpd, v5 = frgcomm, v6 = innovat, v7 = gblsales

TABLE A.29. Global Innovation Model

Paths	Overall	Industrialized	Developing
v3,v1 Economic Env → Mkt/Ind Structure	0.127[a] 0.189[b] .676[c]	.983 .055 17.935	.457 .235 1.929
v3,v2 Regulation → Mkt/Ind Structure	.158 .189 .839	.024 .055 .434	-.070 .235 -.297
v4,v1 Economic Env → Innovation Invst	-.063 .071 -.896	.888 .609 1.468	-.141 .285 -.500
v4,v2 Regulation → Innovation Invst	-.029 .071 -.411	-.041 .112 -.366	-.118 .254 -.467
v4,v3 Mkt/Ind Structure → Innovation Invst	.942 .071 13.157	.043 .612 .071	-.232 .288 -.816
v5,v4 Innovation Invst → Foreign Mkt Invst	.144 .190 .757	-.277 .288 -.957	.559 .221 2.519
v6,v4 Innovation Invst → Global Innovation	.890 .092 9.693	.728 .135 5.372	-.208 .310 -.668
v6,v5 Foreign Mkt Invst → Global Innovation	-.100 .092 -1.089	-.368 .136 -2.720	.303 .311 .972
v7,v6 Global Innovation → Global Sales	.904 .082 11.012	.870 .149 5.849	-.008 .267 -.031
Fit Indices Chi-square; df p-value BBFI BBNFI CFI	28.09;12 0.005 1.000 1.000 1.000	10.842;12 .542 1.000 1.000 1.000	11.20;12 .511 0.991 1.000 1.000

[a] = standardized coefficient, [b] = standard error, [c] = t-value

v1 = pop, v2 = apptime, v3 = mktsize, v4 = r&dexpd, v5 = frgcomm, v6 = innovat, v7 = gblsales

TABLE A.30. Global Innovation Model

Paths	Overall	Industrialized	Developing
v3,v1 Economic Env → Mkt/Ind Structure	0.348[a] 0.180[b] 1.951[c]	.138 .267 .512	.370 .245 1.497
v3,v2 Regulation → Mkt/Ind Structure	.144 .180 .806	.423 .267 1.568	-.099 .245 -.399
v4,v1 Economic Env → Innovation Invst	.136 .199 .686	.949 .106 9.023	-.074 .249 -.300
v4,v2 Regulation → Innovation Invst	.153 .189 .809	.017 .116 .146	-.148 .233 -.638
v4,v3 Mkt/Ind Structure → Innovation Invst	-.229 .199 -1.140	-.133 .118 -1.149	-.468 .253 -1.880
v5,v4 Innovation Invst → Foreign Mkt Invst	.144 .190 .757	-.277 .288 -.957	.559 .221 2.519
v6,v4 Innovation Invst → Global Innovation	.890 .092 9.69	.728 .135 5.374	-.208 .310 -.668
v6,v5 Foreign Mkt Invst → Global Innovation	-.100 .092 -1.089	-.368 .136 -2.720	.303 .311 .972
v7,v6 Global Innovation → Global Sales	.904 .082 11.012	.870 .149 5.850	-.008 .267 -.031
Fit Indices Chi-square; df p-value BBFI BBNFI CFI	35.82;12 0.001 1.000 1.000 1.000	8.947;12 .707 1.000 1.000 1.000	12.63;12 .396 0.991 0.999 1.000

[a] = standardized coefficient, [b] = standard error, [c] = t-value

v1 = pop, v2 = apptime, v3 = mktfocus, v4 = r&dexpd, v5 = frgcomm, v6 = innovat, v7 = gblsales

TABLE A.31. Global Innovation Model

Paths	Overall	Industrialized	Developing
v3,v1 Economic Env → Mkt/Ind Structure	0.046[a] 0.192[b] .238[c]	−.115 .285 −.406	.024 .267 .091
v3,v2 Regulation → Mkt/Ind Structure	.045 .192 .234	.325 .285 1.148	−.033 .267 −.122
v4,v1 Economic Env → Innovation Invst	.058 .191 .305	.941 .109 8.724	−.241 .250 −.971
v4,v2 Regulation → Innovation Invst	.121 .191 .634	−.069 .114 −.606	−.110 .250 −.443
v4,v3 Mkt/Ind Structure → Innovation Invst	−.032 .191 −.168	.090 .114 .786	−.252 .250 −1.015
v5,v4 Innovation Invst → Foreign Mkt Invst	.144 .190 .757	−.277 .288 −.957	.559 .221 2.519
v6,v4 Innovation Invst → Global Innovation	.890 .092 9.693	.728 .135 5.374	−.208 .310 −.668
v6,v5 Foreign Mkt Invst → Global Innovation	−.100 .092 −1.089	−.368 .136 −2.720	.303 .311 .972
v7,v6 Global Innovation → Global Sales	.904 .082 11.012	.870 .149 5.850	−.008 .267 −.031
Fit Indices Chi-square; df p-value BBFI BBNFI CFI	17.52;12 0.131 1.000 1.000 1.000	9.960;12 0.619 1.000 1.000 1.000	10.413;12 .579 1.000 1.000 1.000

[a] = standardized coefficient, [b] = standard error, [c] = t−value

v1 = pop, v2 = apptime, v3 = mktgrwth, v4 = r&dexpd, v5 = frgcomm, v6 = innovat, v7 = gblsales

TABLE A.32. Global Innovation Model

Paths	Overall	Industrialized	Developing
v3,v1 Economic Env → Mkt/Ind Structure	0.095[a] 0.191[b] .498[c]	-.017 .301 -.057	-.021 .264 -.078
v3,v2 Regulation → Mkt/Ind Structure	.066 .191 .347	.064 .301 .214	.148 .264 .561
v4,v1 Economic Env → Innovation Invst	.083 .184 .450	.932 .106 8.839	-.235 .200 -1.180
v4,v2 Regulation → Innovation Invst	.138 .184 .750	-.046 .106 -.437	-.193 .203 -.960
v4,v3 Mkt/Ind Structure → Innovation Invst	-.275 .185 -1.491	.103 .106 .984	.618 .203 3.072
v5,v4 Innovation Invst → Foreign Mkt Invst	.144 .190 .757	-.277 .288 -.957	.559 .221 2.519
v6,v4 Innovation Invst → Global Innovation	.890 .092 9.693	.728 .135 5.373	-.208 .310 -.668
v6,v5 Foreign Mkt Invst → Global Innovation	-.100 .092 -1.089	-.368 .136 -2.720	.303 .311 .972
v7,v6 Global Innovation → Global Sales	.904 .082 11.012	.870 .149 5.849	-.008 .267 -.031
Fit Indices Chi-square; df p-value BBFI BBNFI CFI	16.12;12 0.18 1.000 1.000 1.000	10.455;12 .576 1.000 1.000 1.000	12.44;12 .410 0.997 1.000 1.000

[a] = standardized coefficient, [b] = standard error, [c] = t-value

v1 = pop, v2 = apptime, v3 = mktconc, v4 = r&dexpd, v5 = frgcomm, v6 = innovat, v7 = gblsales

Appendix B

Global Diffusion Models

TABLE B.1. Global Diffusion Model

Paths	Coefficients, Standard Error, t-value
v3,v1 Economic Env → Mkt/Industry Structure	-.167, .287, -.572
v3,v2 Regulation → Mkt/Industry Structure	.192, .287, .658
v4,v1 Economic Env → Market Potential	.503, .187, 2.472
v4,v2 Regulation → Market Potential	-.493, .188, -2.410
v4,v3 Mkt/Industry Structure → Market Potential	.484, .194, 2.336
v5,v4 Market Potential → Incoming Foreign Invst	.582, .259, 2.374
v6,v4 Market Potential → Global Diffusion	-.115, .136, -1.003
v6,v5 Incoming Foreign Invst → Global Diffusion	.035, .129, .306
v6,v7 Global Innovation → Global Diffusion	.946, .102, 10.179
Fit Indices Chi-square; df p-value BBFI BBNFI CFI	8.393;12 .753 .990 1.000 1.000

v1 = gnp, v2 = pricereg, v3 = indfocus, v4 = mktpot, v5 = infrgn, v6 = diff, v7 = innovat

TABLE B.2. Global Diffusion Model

Paths	Coefficients, Standard Error, t-value
v3,v1 Economic Env → Mkt/Industry Structure	-.082, .296, -.275
v3,v2 Regulation → Mkt/Industry Structure	.138, .296, .464
v4,v1 Economic Env → Market Potential	.426, .226, 1.734
v4,v2 Regulation → Market Potential	-.406, .227, -1.643
v4,v3 Mkt/Industry Structure → Market Potential	.046, .229, .186
v5,v4 Market Potential → Incoming Foreign Invst	.582, .259, 2.374
v6,v4 Market Potential → Global Diffusion	-.112, .136, -.976
v6,v5 Incoming Foreign Invst → Global Diffusion	.035, .129, .304
v6,v7 Global Innovation → Global Diffusion	.946, .102, 10.143
Fit Indices Chi-square; df p-value BBFI BBNFI CFI	8.587;12 .737 .999 1.000 1.000

v1 = gnp, v2 = pricereg, v3 = indgrwth, v4 = mktpot, v5 = infrgn, v6 = diff, v7 = innovat

TABLE B.3. Global Diffusion Model

Paths	Coefficients, Standard Error, t-value
v3,v1 Economic Env → Mkt/Industry Structure	-.067, .284, .234
v3,v2 Regulation → Mkt/Industry Structure	-.301, .284, -1.048
v4,v1 Economic Env → Market Potential	.434, .221, 1.807
v4,v2 Regulation → Market Potential	-.454, .231, -1.805
v4,v3 Mkt/Industry Structure → Market Potential	-.180, .234, -.713
v5,v4 Market Potential → Incoming Foreign Invst	.582, .259, 2.374
v6,v4 Market Potential → Global Diffusion	-.104, .137, -.905
v6,v5 Incoming Foreign Invst → Global Diffusion	.034, .129, .297
v6,v7 Global Innovation → Global Diffusion	.946, .102, 10.088
Fit Indices Chi-square; df p-value BBFI BBNFI CFI	9.636;12 .647 1.000 1.000 1.000

v1 = gnp, v2 = pricereg, v3 = indconc, v4 = mktpot, v5 = infrgn, v6 = diff, v7 = innovat

TABLE B.4. Global Diffusion Model

Paths	Coefficients, Standard Error, t-value
v3,v1 Economic Env → Mkt/Industry Structure	-.332, .252, -1.306
v3,v2 Regulation → Mkt/Industry Structure	.476, .252, 1.928
v4,v1 Economic Env → Market Potential	.721, .231, 3.092
v4,v2 Regulation → Market Potential	-.081, .249, -.321
v4,v3 Mkt/Industry Structure → Market Potential	.442, .257, 1.668
v5,v4 Market Potential → Incoming Foreign Invst	.611, .240, 2.561
v6,v4 Market Potential → Global Diffusion	-.112, .130, -.949
v6,v5 Incoming Foreign Invst → Global Diffusion	.035, .129, .297
v6,v7 Global Innovation → Global Diffusion	.946, .102, 10.090
Fit Indices Chi-square; df p-value BBFI BBNFI CFI	6.426;12 .893 .990 1.000 1.000

v1 = gnp, v2 = apptime, v3 = indfocus, v4 = mktpot, v5 = infrgn, v6 = diff, v7 = innovat

TABLE B.5. Global Diffusion Model

Paths	Coefficients, Standard Error, t-value
v3,v1 Economic Env → Mkt/Industry Structure	-.197, .281, -.706
v3,v2 Regulation → Mkt/Industry Structure	.329, .281, 1.180
v4,v1 Economic Env → Market Potential	.570, .246, 2.299
v4,v2 Regulation → Market Potential	.144, .255, .558
v4,v3 Mkt/Industry Structure → Market Potential	-.042, .258, -.161
v5,v4 Market Potential → Incoming Foreign Invst	.611, .240, 2.561
v6,v4 Market Potential → Global Diffusion	-.139, .130, -1.216
v6,v5 Incoming Foreign Invst → Global Diffusion	.037, .129, .323
v6,v7 Global Innovation → Global Diffusion	.946, .102, 10.441
Fit Indices Chi-square; df p-value BBFI BBNFI CFI	7.848;12 .796 .990 1.000 1.000

v1 = gnp, v2 = apptime, v3 = indgrwth, v4 = mktpot, v5 = infrgn, v6 = diff, v7 = innovat

TABLE B.6. Global Diffusion Model

Paths	Coefficients, Standard Error, t-value
v3,v1 Economic Env → Mkt/Industry Structure	.225, .293, .768
v3,v2 Regulation → Mkt/Industry Structure	.033, .293, .113
v4,v1 Economic Env → Market Potential	.597, .246, 2.405
v4,v2 Regulation → Market Potential	.132, .240, .548
v4,v3 Mkt/Industry Structure → Market Potential	-.081, .246, -.325
v5,v4 Market Potential → Incoming Foreign Invst	.611, .240, 2.561
v6,v4 Market Potential → Global Diffusion	-.147, .130, -1.298
v6,v5 Incoming Foreign Invst → Global Diffusion	.038, .129, .331
v6,v7 Global Innovation → Global Diffusion	.946, .102, 10.551
Fit Indices Chi-square; df p-value BBFI BBNFI CFI	8.265;12 .764 1.000 1.000 1.000

v1 = gnp, v2 = apptime, v3 = indconc, v4 = mktpot, v5 = infrgn, v6 = diff, v7 = innovat

TABLE B.7. Global Diffusion Model

Paths	Coefficients, Standard Error, t-value
v3,v1 Economic Env → Mkt/Industry Structure	.502, .250, 2.455
v3,v2 Regulation → Mkt/Industry Structure	.536, .250, 2.618
v4,v1 Economic Env → Market Potential	1.002, .067, 15.281
v4,v2 Regulation → Market Potential	.054, .069, .811
v4,v3 Mkt/Industry Structure → Market Potential	-.036, .065, -.461
v5,v4 Market Potential → Incoming Foreign Invst	.623, .233, 2.641
v6,v4 Market Potential → Global Diffusion	-.134, .127, -1.147
v6,v5 Incoming Foreign Invst → Global Diffusion	.037, .129, .314
v6,v7 Global Innovation → Global Diffusion	.946, .102, 10.322
Fit Indices Chi-square; df p-value BBFI BBNFI CFI	9.387;12 .669 1.000 1.000 1.000

v1 = pop, v2 = pricereg, v3 = infocus, v4 = mktpot, v5 = infrgn, v6 = diff, v7 = innovat

TABLE B.8. Global Diffusion Model

Paths	Coefficients, Standard Error, t–value
v3,v1 Economic Env → Mkt/Industry Structure	-.087, .296, .297
v3,v2 Regulation → Mkt/Industry Structure	.233, .296, .797
v4,v1 Economic Env → Market Potential	.987, .053, 18.880
v4,v2 Regulation → Market Potential	.044, .055, .821
v4,v3 Mkt/Industry Structure → Market Potential	-.037, .054, -.695
v5,v4 Market Potential → Incoming Foreign Invst	.623, .233, 2.641
v6,v4 Market Potential → Global Diffusion	-.131, .127, -1.119
v6,v5 Incoming Foreign Invst → Global Diffusion	.037, .129, .311
v6,v7 Global Innovation → Global Diffusion	.946, .102, 10.285
Fit Indices Chi-square; df p–value BBFI BBNFI CFI	8.131;12 .774 1.000 1.000 1.000

v1 = pop, v2 = pricereg, v3 = indgrwth, v4 = mktpot, v5 = infrgn, v6 = diff, v7 = innovat

TABLE B.9. Global Diffusion Model

Paths	Coefficients, Standard Error, t-value
v3,v1 Economic Env → Mkt/Industry Structure	-.304, .273, -1.233
v3,v2 Regulation → Mkt/Industry Structure	-.488, .273, -1.979
v4,v1 Economic Env → Market Potential	1.016, .050, 20.656
v4,v2 Regulation → Market Potential	.088, .055, 1.633
v4,v3 Mkt/Industry Structure → Market Potential	.107, .052, 1.906
v5,v4 Market Potential → Incoming Foreign Invst	.623, .233, 2.641
v6,v4 Market Potential → Global Diffusion	-.134, .127, -1.146
v6,v5 Incoming Foreign Invst → Global Diffusion	.037, .129, .314
v6,v7 Global Innovation → Global Diffusion	.946, .102, 10.326
Fit Indices Chi-square; df p-value BBFI BBNFI CFI	9.724;12 .6401 1.000 1.000 1.000

v1 = pop, v2 = pricereg, v3 = indconc, v4 = mktpot, v5 = infrgn, v6 = diff,
v7 = innovat

TABLE B.10. Global Diffusion Model

Paths	Coefficients, Standard Error, t-value
v3,v1 Economic Env → Mkt/Industry Structure	.138, .267, .511
v3,v2 Regulation → Mkt/Industry Structure	.423, .267, 1.569
v4,v1 Economic Env → Market Potential	.986, .055, 17.856
v4,v2 Regulation → Market Potential	.032, .060, .532
v4,v3 Mkt/Industry Structure → Market Potential	-.020, .061, -.321
v5,v4 Market Potential → Incoming Foreign Invst	.613, .239, 2.574
v6,v4 Market Potential → Global Diffusion	-.148, .129, -1.305
v6,v5 Incoming Foreign Invst → Global Diffusion	.038, .129, .331
v6,v7 Global Innovation → Global Diffusion	.946, .102, 10.547
Fit Indices Chi-square; df p-value BBFI BBNFI CFI	6.223;12 .904 1.000 1.000 1.000

v1 = pop, v2 = apptime, v3 = indfocus, v4 = mktpot, v5 = infrgn, v6 = diff, v7 = innovat

TABLE B.11. Global Diffusion Model

Paths	Coefficients, Standard Error, t-value
v3,v1 Economic Env → Mkt/Industry Structure	-.115, .285, -.406
v3,v2 Regulation → Mkt/Industry Structure	.325, .285, 1.148
v4,v1 Economic Env → Market Potential	.978, .054, 18.176
v4,v2 Regulation → Market Potential	.038, .056, .672
v4,v3 Mkt/Industry Structure → Market Potential	-.044, .056, -.765
v5,v4 Market Potential → Incoming Foreign Invst	.613, .239, 2.574
v6,v4 Market Potential → Global Diffusion	-.149, .129, -1.297
v6,v5 Incoming Foreign Invst → Global Diffusion	.038, .129, .330
v6,v7 Global Innovation → Global Diffusion	.945, .102, 10.405
Fit Indices Chi-square; df p-value BBFI BBNFI CFI	6.753;12 .873 1.000 1.000 1.000

v1 = pop, v2 = apptime, v3 = indgrwth, v4 = mktpot, v5 = infrgn, v6 = diff, v7 = innovat

TABLE B.12. Global Diffusion Model

Paths	Coefficients, Standard Error, t-value
v3,v1 Economic Env → Mkt/Industry Structure	-.017, .301, -.057
v3,v2 Regulation → Mkt/Industry Structure	.065, .301, .215
v4,v1 Economic Env → Market Potential	.984, .051, 19.360
v4,v2 Regulation → Market Potential	.019, .051, .381
v4,v3 Mkt/Industry Structure → Market Potential	.068, .051, 1.339
v5,v4 Market Potential → Incoming Foreign Invst	.613, .239, 2.574
v6,v4 Market Potential → Global Diffusion	-.153, .129, -1.341
v6,v5 Incoming Foreign Invst → Global Diffusion	.038, .129, .335
v6,v7 Global Innovation → Global Diffusion	.945, .102, 10.460
Fit Indices Chi-square; df p-value BBFI BBNFI CFI	7.107;12 .8504 1.000 1.000 1.000

v1 = pop, v2 = apptime, v3 = indconc, v4 = mktpot, v5 = infrgn, v6 = diff, v7 = innovat

Notes

Preface

1. An "ethical" pharmaceutical is one that is available only through prescription. Ethical products can be either patented or nonpatented (i.e., generic).
2. An NCE is a drug for which the active ingredient has not been previously marketed (approved) for use in a drug product.

Chapter 1

1. See Smith (1983) for a review.
2. Thalidomide was a tranquilizer-sedative marketed by Chemie Grunenthal in West Germany as a nonprescription drug. The product was distributed for approximately three years before Dr. Leng, a pediatrician at the University of Hamburg, discovered and reported to the company that it caused phocomelia, a birth defect in infants. By this time, several thousand infants had been affected.
3. A globally successful NCE or global NCE is defined as an NCE that has been approved/marketed in at least seven of the major pharmaceutical country markets, i.e., France, Germany, Japan, Italy, Switzerland, the United Kingdom, and the United States.

Chapter 2

1. Following the thalidomide tragedy, the U.S. Congress passed the Kefauver-Harris Amendments. This extended the mandate and regulatory control of the FDA in several ways:

  • It required firms to provide documented scientific evidence of a new drug's efficacy, in addition to the proof of safety required by the original law.
  • It gave the FDA, for the first time, discretionary power over the clinical research process. Thus, prior to any tests on human beings, firms are now required to submit a new drug investigational plan (IND), giving the results of animal tests and research protocols for human tests.

2. NCEs are classified by the FDA into three categories: (1) drugs offering little or no gain, (2) drugs offering modest gain, and (3) drugs offering important gains.

Chapter 4

1. Group A—Countries with a sophisticated pharmaceutical industry and a significant research base, Group B—Countries with innovative capabilities, Group C—Countries with reproductive capabilities, and Group D—Countries without a pharmaceutical industry.

Bibliography

Adams, I. and L. Klein (Eds.) (1982). *Industrial Policies for Growth and Competitiveness: An Economic Perspective*, Lexington, MA: D.C. Heath.

Agrawal, M. (1993). "International Pharmaceutical Marketing: An Historical Perspective." In *Proceedings of the Sixth Conference on Historical Research in Marketing and Marketing Thought*, Jeffrey B. Schmidt, Stanley C. Hollander, Terence Nevett, and Jagdish N. Sheth (Eds.), Ann Arbor, MI: Michigan State University, 363-376.

Ballance, R., J. Pogany, and H. Forstner (1992). *The World's Pharmaceutical Industries: An International Perspective on Innovation, Competition and Policy*, Aldershot, England: Edward Elgar Publishing Ltd.

Bogner, W.C. and H. Thomas (1992). *Core Competence and Competitive Advantage: A Model and Illustrative Evidence from the Pharmaceutical Industry*, WP 4900, no-92-0174, University of Illinois at Urbana-Champaign: Bureau of Economic and Business Research.

Bolton, M.K. and N.A. Boyacigiller (1993). "A Model for Comparative Research on New Product Introductions." In *Advances in International Comparative Management*, 8, 217-240.

Brownlee, O.H. (1979). "The Economic Consequences of Regulating without Regard to Economic Consequences." In *Issues in Pharmaceutical Economics*, Robert I. Chien (Ed.). Lexington, MA: D.C. Heath, 215-228.

Business Week (1990). "Japan's Next Battleground: The Medicine Chest." (March 12), 68.

Carre, J.J., P. Dubois, and E. Malinvaud (1975). *French Economic Growth*, Stanford, CA: Stanford University Press.

Caves, R.E., M.D. Whinston, and M.A. Hurwitz (1991). "Patent Expiration, Entry, and Competition in the U.S. Pharmaceutical Industry." In *Brookings Papers: Microeconomics*, Washington, DC: Brookings Institute, 1-66.

Chemical Engineering News (1961). "Britain's Drug Makers Under Fire." 39, (March 6), 92-93.

Chemical Marketing Reporter (1991). "Drug Producers in U.S. Find Overseas Rivals a Challenge." 240, (July 29), 7-8.

Chemical Marketing Reporter (1992a). "Pharmaceuticals '92: Legislative Incisions." 241(10), (March 9), SR6-SR8.

Chemical Marketing Reporter (1992b). "Pharmaceuticals '92: To Cap or Not to Cap." 241(10), (March 9), SR3-SR4.

Chemical Week (1991). "Pharmaceuticals: Pressure on Prices and Profits." 149(2), (August 7), 26-31.

Clymer, H.A. (1970). "The Changing Costs of Pharmaceutical Innovation." In *Proceedings of the First Seminar on Economics of Pharmaceutical Innovation*, Joseph D. Cooper (Ed.). Washington, DC: The American University, 109-124.

Clymer, H.A. (1975). "The Economic and Regulatory Climate: U.S. and Overseas Trends." In *Drug Development and Marketing,* Robert B. Helms (Ed.). Washington, DC: American Enterprise Institute for Public Policy Research, 137-154.

Cohen, S., D. Teece, L. Tyson, and J. Zysman (1984). "Global Competition, The New Reality." *Working paper of the President's Commission on Industrial Competitiveness*, Berkeley, CA: University of California.

Comanor, W.S. (1986). "The Political Economy of the Pharmaceutical Industry." *Journal of Economic Literature*, 24, (September), 1178-1217.

Commission on Industrial Competitiveness (1985). *Global Competition: The New Reality*, Berkeley, CA: University of California.

Cooper, J.D. (1969). "The Economics of Drug Innovation." In *Proceedings of the First Seminar on Economics of Pharmaceutical Innovation*, Joseph D. Cooper (Ed.). Washington, DC: The American University.

Cooper, J.D. (1976). "Regulation, Economics, and Pharmaceutical Innovation." In *Proceedings of the First Seminar on Economics of Pharmaceutical Innovation,* Joseph D. Cooper (Ed.). Washington, DC: The American University.

Cornwall, J. (1976). "Diffusion, Convergence, and Kaldor's Law." *Economic Journal*, 85, 307-314.

Council on Competitiveness (1991). *A Competitive Profile of the Drugs and Pharmaceutical Industry*, Washington, DC: Council on Competitiveness.

Davis, L.A. (1991). "Technology Intensity of U.S., Canadian, and Japanese Manufacturers Output and Exports." In *Technology and National Competitiveness: Oligopoly, Technological Innovation, and International Competition*, Jorge Niosi (Ed.). Montreal: McGill-Queens University Press.

Dension, E.F. (1967). *Why Growth Rates Differ: Post-War Experience in Nine Western Countries*, Washington, DC: Brookings Institute.

DiMasi, J., R. Hansen, H. Grabowski, and L. Lasagna (1991). "The Cost of Innovation in the Pharmaceutical Industry." *Journal of Health Economics*, 10(2), 107-142.

Dixit, A. (1986). "Trade Policy: An Agenda for Research." In *Strategic Trade Policy and the New International Economics*, P. Krugman (Ed.). Boston, MA: MIT Press.

Dosi, G. and L. Soete (1991). "Technological Innovation and International Competitiveness." In *Technology and National Competitiveness: Oligopoly, Technological Innovation, and International Competition,* Jorge Niosi (Ed.). Montreal: McGill-Queens University Press.

Dunning, J.H. (1988). "International Direct Investment in Innovation: The Pharmaceutical Industry." In *Multinationals, Technology, and Competitiveness*, London: Unwin Hyman, 123-141.

The Economist (1986). "Drugs in Asia: Opening a New Medicine Chest." 299(7448) (May 31).

The Economist (1988). "Selling to Japan: Drug on the Market." 309 (December 10), 70.

The Economist (1989). "The New World of Drugs." 310(7588), (February 4), 63.

Ernst, D. and D. O'Connor (1989). *Technology and Global Competition: The Challenge for Newly Industrializing Economies,* Washington, DC: OECD.

European Chemical News (1989). "Pharmaceutical Pricing: A Cause for French Concern." March 20, 20.

Fagerberg, J. (1987). "A Technology Gap Approach to Why Growth Rates Differ." In *The Economics of Innovation,* Christopher Freeman (Ed.). Aldershot, England: Edward Elgar Pub. Ltd., 55-67.

Fenton, R.C. (1963). "Worldwide Ethical Drug Markets." *Drug and Cosmetic Industry,* 93, (November), 624.

Financial World (1989). "Pharmaceuticals." 158, (May 30), 53-80.

Franko, L.G. (1987). "Global Competitive Performance and the Geographic Location of Corporate Activity." Presented at the *Strategic Management Society Conference,* Boston.

Franko, L.G. (1989). "Global Corporate Competition: Who's Winning, Who's Losing, and the R&D Factor as One Reason Why." *Strategic Management Journal,* 10, 449-474.

Geringer, M.J. and P.W. Beamish (1989). "Diversification Strategy and Internationalization: Implications for MNE Performance." *Strategic Management Journal,* 10, 109-119.

Ghoshal, S. (1987). "Global Strategy: An Organizing Framework." *Strategic Management Journal,* 8(5), 425-440.

Goldstein, J. and S. Krasner (1984). "Unfair Trade Practices: The Case for a Differential Response." *American Economic Review,* 74(2), 282-287.

Gomulka, S. (1971). "Inventive Activity, Diffusion and Stages of Economic Growth." *Skrifter fra Aarhus Universitets Okonomiske Institut* nr. 24, Aarhus, Denmark.

Grabowski, H.G. (1976). "Structural Effects of Regulation in the Ethical Drug Industry." In *Drug Regulation and Innovation: Empirical Evidence and Policy Options,* Washington, DC: American Enterprise Institute for Public Policy Research, 55-63.

Grabowski, H.G. (1980). "Regulation and the International Diffusion of Pharmaceuticals." In *The International Supply of Medicines,* Robert B. Helms (Ed.). Washington, DC: American Enterprise Institute for Public Policy Research.

Grabowski, H.G. (1989). "An Analysis of U.S. International Competitiveness in Pharmaceuticals." *Managerial and Decision Economics,* Special Issue, 27-33.

Grabowski, H.G. (1990). "Innovation and International Competitiveness in Pharmaceuticals." In *The Proceedings of the 2nd International Joseph Schumpeter Society Meetings,* Ann Arbor, MI: University of Michigan, 167-185.

Grabowski, H.G. and L.G. Thomas (1978). "Estimating the Effects of Regulation on Innovation: An International Comparative Analysis of the Pharmaceutical Industry." *Journal of Law and Economics,* 21(1), Spring, 133-163.

Grabowski, H.G. and J.M. Vernon (1976). "Structural Effects of Regulation on Innovation in the Ethical Drug Industry." In *Essays on Industrial Organization in Honor of Joe Bain*, R. Masson and D. Qualls (Eds.). Cambridge, MA: Ballinger.

Grabowski, H.G. and J.M. Vernon (1977). "Consumer Protection Regulation in Ethical Drugs." *American Economic Review*, 67, (February), 359-364.

Grant, R.M. (1987). "Multinationality and Performance Among British Manufacturing Companies." *Journal of International Business Studies*, 18(3), 79-89.

Hamel, G., Y.L. Doz, and C.K. Prahalad (1989). "Collaborate with Your Competitors and Win." *Harvard Business Review*, (January/February), 133-139.

Hansen, R (1979). "The Pharmaceutical Development Process: Estimates of Development Costs and Times and the Effects of Proposed Regulatory Changes." In *Issues in Pharmaceutical Economics*, R. Chien (Ed.). Lexington, MA: Lexington Books.

Harberger, A.C. (Ed.) (1984). *World Economic Growth*, San Francisco, CA: ICS Press.

Harrigan, K.R. (1987). "Strategic Alliances: Their New Role in Global Competition." *Columbia Journal of World Business*, (Summer), 67-69.

Hatsopoulos, G., P. Krugman, and L. Summers (1988). "U.S. Competitiveness: Beyond the Trade Deficit." *Science*, 241(4863), (July 15), p. 299.

Hatzichronoglou, T. (1991). "Indicators of Industrial Competitiveness: Results and Limitations." In *Technology and National Competitiveness: Oligopoly, Technological Innovation, and International Competition*, Jorge Niosi (Ed.). Montreal: McGill-Queens University Press.

Hauptman, O. and E.B. Roberts (1987). "FDA Regulation of Product Risk and Its Impact Upon Young Biomedical Firms." *Journal of Product Innovation Management*, 4(2), (June), 138-148.

Hayduk, L.A. (1987). *Structural Equation Modeling with Lisrel: Essentials and Advances*, Baltimore: John Hopkins University Press.

Howe, D.C. (1992). "Pharmaceuticals in Southeast Asia: Markets, Production and Competitors: Part I." *East Asian Executive Reports*, 14(11), (November 15), 8, 22-25.

——— (1993). ""Pharmaceuticals in Southeast Asia: Markets, Production and Competitors: Part II." *East Asian Executive Reports*, 15(1), (January 15), 8-24.

Huber, P. (1988). *Liability: The Legal Revolution and its Consequences*, New York: Basic Books.

Hymer, S.H. (1960). *The International Operations of National Firms: A Study of Direct Foreign Investment*, PhD Dissertation, Boston, MA: MIT.

The IMS World Drug Market Manual (Asia), 1990. Copyright IMSWorld Publications Limited, London, U.K.

ITA (International Trade Administration) (1984). *A Competitive Assessment of the U.S. Pharmaceutical Industry*, Washington, DC: U.S. Department of Commerce.

Jaffe, M.E. (1976). "Drug Regulatory Patterns Worldwide: Trends and Realities." In *Impact of Public Policy on Drug Innovation and Pricing*, S.A. Mitchell and E.A. Link (Eds.). Washington, DC: The American University, 277-287.

Jaffe, T. (1983). "Drugs." *Forbes*, 131, (January 3), 192-193.

James, B.G. (1983). "International Marketing." In *Principles of Pharmaceutical Marketing,*" Third Edition, Mickey C. Smith (Ed.). Philadelphia: Lea and Febiger.

The Japan Times (1990). "Japan Patents Wrapped in Red Tape." August 27, 20.

Jarrell, S. (1983). "Research and Development and Firm Size in the Pharmaceutical Industry." *Business Economics,* (September), 26-39.

Johnson, C. (Ed.) (1984). *The Industrial Policy Debate,* Washington, DC: Institute for Contemporary Studies.

Kamien, M.I. and N.L. Schwartz (1970). "Market Structure, Elasticity of Demand and the Incentive to Invest." *Journal of Law and Economics,* 13(1).

Kamien, M.I. and N.L. Schwartz (1982). *Market Structure and Innovation,* New York: Cambridge University Press.

Keller, B.G. and M.C. Smith (1969). *Pharmaceutical Marketing: An Anthology and Bibliography.* Baltimore: The Williams and Wilkins Co.

Kennedy, P.M. (1987). *The Rise and Fall of the Great Powers: Economic Change and Military Conflict from 1500 to 2000,* New York: Random House.

Kochhar, R. and M.A. Hitt (1995). "Toward an Integrative Model of International Diversification." *Journal of International Management,* 1(1), 33-72.

Kogut, B. (1985). "Designing Global Strategies: Comparative and Competitive Value-Added Chains." *Sloan Management Review,* (Summer), 15-28.

Kremers, E. and G. Urdang (1940). *History of Pharmacy: A Guide and a Survey.* Philadelphia: J.B. Lippincott Co.

LaFrancis-Popper, K.M. and R.W. Nason (1994). "The Drug Lag: A 20-Year Analysis of Six Country Markets." *Journal of Public Policy and Marketing,* 13(2), (Fall), 290-299.

Lall, S. (1985). "Appropriate Pharmaceutical Policies in Developing Countries." *Managerial and Decision Economics,* 6(4).

———— (1990). *Building Industrial Competitiveness in Developing Countries,* Paris: OECD.

Landau, R. (1990). "Capital Investment: Key to Competitiveness and Growth." *The Brookings Review,* 8(3), Summer.

Lasagna, L. (1969). "Constraints on the Innovation of Drugs." In *Proceedings of the First Seminar on Economics of Pharmaceutical Innovation,* Joseph D. Cooper (Ed.). Washington, DC: The American University.

———— (1989). "Congress, the FDA, and New Drug Development: Before and After 1962." *Perspectives in Biology and Medicine,* 32(3), Spring.

———— (1991). "The Chilling Effect of Product Liability on New Drug Development." In *The Liability Maze,* Peter W. Huber and Robert E. Litan (Eds.). Washington, DC: The Brookings Institute, 334-359.

Lasagna, L. and W.M. Wardell (1975). "The Rate of New Drug Discovery." In *Drug Development and Marketing,* Robert B. Helms (Ed.). Washington, DC: American Enterprise Institute for Public Policy Research, 137-154.

Leonard, W.N. (1971). "Research and Development in Industrial Growth." *Journal of Political Economy,* 79(2), (March/April), 232-256.

Longman, R. (1994). "Joint Marketing in Europe." *Pharmaceutical Strategic Alliances*, Fourth Edition, Norwalk, CT: Windhover Information Inc.

Loury, G.C. (1979). "Market Structure and Innovation." *Quarterly Journal of Economics*, August.

Magaziner, I. and R. Reich (1982). *Minding America's Business*, Orlando, FL: Harcourt Brace Jovanovich.

Mansfield, E. (1968). *Industrial Research and Technological Innovation*, New York: W.W. Norton.

Medical Advertising Newsletter (1990). September 15, 4-5.

Medical Marketing (1990). "Japan: The Pharmaceutical Market Here Is the World's 2nd Largest." August. 22-34.

Merck and Co. (1988). *Health Care Innovation: The Case for a Favorable Public Policy*, 23.

Mitchell, S.A. and E.A. Link (Eds.) (1976). *Impact of Public Policy on Drug Innovation and Pricing*, Washington, DC: The American University.

Moskowitz, M. (1961). "Drugs, the International Explosion." *Drug and Cosmetic Industry*, 88, (January), 42.

NAE (1983). *The Competitive Status of the U.S. Pharmaceutical Industry: The Influences of Technology in Determining Industrial Competitive Advantage*, Washington, DC: National Academy Press.

Narayana, P.L. (1984). *The Indian Pharmaceutical Industry: Problems and Prospects*, New Delhi, India: NCAER.

Niosi, J. (1991). *Technology and National Competitiveness: Oligopoly, Technological Innovation, and International Competition*, Jorge Niosi (Ed.). Montreal: McGill-Queens University Press.

Niosi, J. and P. Faucher (1991). "The State and International Trade: Technology and Competitiveness." In *Technology and National Competitiveness: Oligopoly, Technological Innovation, and International Competition,* J. Niosi (Ed.), Montreal: McGill-Queens University Press, 119-141.

Ohmae, K. (1989). "The Global Logic of Strategic Alliances." *Harvard Business Review,* (March/April), 143-154.

Parker, J.E.S. (1984). *The International Diffusion of Pharmaceuticals*, New York: St. Martin's Press.

Peltzman, S. (1973). "An Evaluation of Consumer Protection Legislation: The 1962 Drug Amendments." *Journal of Political Economy*, 81, (September/October), 1049-1091.

Peltzman, S., J. DiRaddo, and A. Fringeri (1980). "A Preliminary Analysis of the Rate of Development of New Drugs by British-Owned Pharmaceutical Firms." In *Proceedings of a Symposium on Risk and Regulation,* London: Trust for Education and Research in Therapeutics.

Peltzman, S., M. May, and G. Trimble (1982). "New Drug Development by United States Pharmaceutical Firms." *Clinical Pharmacology and Therapeutics,* 32, 407-417.

Phillips, A. (1956). "Concentration, Scale and Technological Change in Selected Manufacturing Industries, 1899-1939." *Journal of Industrial Economics*, June.

PMA (1989). *PMA Facts at a Glance*, Washington, DC: Pharmaceutical Manufacturers Association, 7.

PMA (1990). Better Health Through New Medicines and an Improved FDA, Statement to the Subcommittee on Drugs and Biologics of the Advisory Committee on the Food and Drug Administration, Department of Health and Human Services, September 13, Washington, DC: Pharmaceutical Manufacturers Association, 1-5.

Porter, M.E. (1990). *The Competitive Advantage of Nations*, New York: Free Press.

Posner, M.V. (1961). "International Trade and Technical Change." *Oxford Economic Papers*, 13, 323-341.

Pradhan, S.B. (1983). *International Pharmaceutical Marketing*, Westport, CT: Quorum Books.

Prahalad, C.K. and G. Hamel (1990). "The Core Competence of the Corporation." *Harvard Business Review*, (May-June), 79-91.

Redwood, H. (1988). *The Pharmaceutical Industry—Trends, Problems, and Achievements*, England: Oldwicks Press Ltd.

———— (1991). "Pharmaceuticals: The Price/Research Spiral." *Long Range Planning*, 24(2), (April), 16-27.

Reich, R. (1983). "Beyond Free Trade." *Foreign Affairs*, 61:4.

Robinson, R.D. (1991). "Toward Creating an International Technology Transfer Paradigm." In *The International Communication of Technology: A Book of Readings*, Richard D. Robinson (Ed.). New York: Taylor and Francis.

Rothwell, R. and W. Zegveld (1981). "Government Regulations and Innovation." In *Industrial Innovation and Public Policy: Preparing for the 1980s and the 1990s*, Westport, CT: Greenwood Press.

Rugman, A. (1985). "National Strategies for International Competitiveness." *Multinational Business*, (3), 1-9.

Sarett, L.H. (1974). "FDA Regulations and Their Influence on Future R&D." *Research Management*, 27, (March), 18-20.

Schankerman, M. (1976). "Common Costs in Pharmaceutical Research and Development: Implications for Direct Price Regulation." In *Impact of Public Policy on Drug Innovation and Pricing*, S.A. Mitchell and E.A. Link (Eds.). Washington, DC: The American University.

Scherer, F.M. (1976). "Corporate Inventive Output, Profits, and Growth." *Journal of Political Economy*, 73(3), (December), 101-111.

Schumpeter, J. (1934). *The Theory of Economic Development*, Cambridge, MA: Harvard University Press.

Schwartzman, D. (1976). *Innovation in the Pharmaceutical Industry*, Baltimore: Johns Hopkins University Press.

Scott, R.S. and G.C. Lodge (1985). *U.S. Competitiveness in the World Economy*, Boston, MA: Harvard Business School Press.

Scrip (1990). "Prospects for 'Bungyo' in Japan." April 27, p. 26.

Scrip League Tables (1989). PJB Pubs. Ltd., UK.

Scrip Magazine (1994). "Single-Digit Growth for World Pharmaceutical Market." PJB Pubs. Ltd., UK.

Scrip Magazine (1997). "Scrip's Review of 1996." PJB Publications Ltd., Sussex, UK.

Scrip Magazine (1998). "Scrip's Review of 1997." PJB Publications Ltd., Sussex, UK.

Scrip Review (1990). PJB Publications Ltd., Sussex, UK.

Scrip Review (1991). PJB Publications Ltd., Sussex, UK

Shan, W. and W. Hamilton (1991). "Country-Specific Advantage and International Cooperation." *Strategic Management Journal*, 12, 419-432.

Smith, M.C.(1983). *Principles of Pharmaceutical Marketing*, Third Edition, Mickey C. Smith (Ed.). Philadelphia: Lea and Febiger.

————— (1991). *Pharmaceutical Marketing: Strategy and Cases*, Binghamton, NY: The Haworth Press, Inc.

Spilker, B. (1989). *Multinational Drug Companies: Issues in Drug Discovery and Development*, New York: Raven Press.

Steward, H.F. (1977). "Public Policy and Innovation in the Drug Industry." In *Providing for Health Services*, Sir Douglas Black and G.P. Thomas (Eds.). London: Croom Helm.

Swazey, J.P. (1991). "Prescription Drug Safety and Product Liability." In *The Liability Maze*, Peter W. Huber and Robert E. Litan (Eds.). Washington, DC: The Brookings Institute, 291-333.

Taggart, J.H. (1993). *The World Pharmaceutical Industry*, London: Routledge.

Takada, H. and D. Jain (1991). "Cross-National Analysis of Diffusion of Consumer Durable Goods in Pacific Rim Countries." *Journal of Marketing*, 55, (April), 48-54.

Temin, P. (1979). "Technology, Regulation, and Market Structure in the Modern Pharmaceutical Industry." *Bell Journal of Economics*, 10, (Autumn), 427-446.

Temple, P. (1991). "Tougher Times Ahead for a Global Market." *Accountancy*, 107, (February), 88-89.

Thomas, H. and R.M. Grant (1987). "Is Diversification Profitable?" Presented at *Strategic Management Society Conference*, Boston.

Thomas, L.G. (1989). "Spare the Rod and Spoil the Industry: Vigorous Competition and Vigorous Regulation Promote Global Competitive Advantages." Unpublished, October.

————— (1990). "Regulation and Firm Size: FDA Impacts on Innovation." *Rand Journal of Economics,* 21(4), (Winter), 497-517.

Thorelli, H.B. (1990). "International Marketing: An Ecologic View." In *International Marketing Strategy*, Third Edition, Hans B. Thorelli and S. Tamer Cavusgil (Eds.). New York: Pergamon Press.

Tokyo Business Today (1988). "No Magic Pill for Pharmaceutical Makers." (June), 34-38.

Tokyo Business Today (1990). "Japanese Pharmaceutical Makers Are Globalizing Operations." (June), 34-35.

Toyne, B. and P.G.P. Walters (1993). "Global Business Operations: Patterns and Theories." In *Global Marketing Management: A Strategic Perspective*, Second Edition, Boston: Allyn and Bacon.

Tyson, L. (1990). "Managed Trade: Making the Best of Second Best." In *An American Trade Strategy: Options for the 1990s*, R. Lawrence and C. Shultze (Eds.). Washington, DC: Brookings Institute.

U.S. Department of Commerce (1989). *U.S. Direct Investment Abroad: Operations of U.S. Parent Companies and their Foreign Affiliates*, July 1989, Washington, DC: Author.

U.S. Industrial Outlook (1991). *Drugs*, p. 45-2.

USITC (1990). "Japan's Distribution System and Options for Improving U.S. Access." *USITC Publication 2327*, October, 2-11.

USITC (1991). *Global Competitiveness of U.S. Advanced-Technology Manufacturing Industries: Pharmaceuticals*, Washington, DC: United States International Trade Commission.

Villard, H.H. (1958). "Competition, Oligopoly and Research." *Journal of Political Economy*, December.

Wachter, M. and S. Wachter (Eds.) (1982). *Toward a New U.S. Industrial Policy*, Philadelphia, PA: University of Pennsylvania.

Wardell, W.M. (1973). "Introduction of New Therapeutic Drugs in the U.S. and Great Britain: An International Comparison." *Clinical Pharmacology and Therapeutics*, 14(5), (September-October), 773-790.

_____ (1974). "Therapeutic Implications of the Drug Lag." *Clinical Pharmacology and Therapeutics*, 15(1) (January), 73-96.

_____ (1975). "Developments in the Introduction of New Drugs in the United States and Great Britain, 1971-1974." In *Drug Development and Marketing*, Robert B. Helms (Ed.). Washington, DC: American Enterprise Institute for Public Policy Research, 165-182.

Wardell, W.M. and L.E. Sheck (1982). "Is Pharmaceutical Innovation Declining? Interpreting Measures of Pharmaceutical Innovation and Regulatory Impact in the USA, 1950-1980." In *Pharmaceutical Economics*, Bjorn Lindgren (Ed.). Stockholm: Swedish Institute for Health Economics, 177-189.

Wiggins, S.N. (1981). "Product Quality Regulation and New Drug Introductions: Some New Evidence from the 1970s." *Review of Economics and Statistics*, 63, 615-619.

_____ (1983). "The Impact of Regulation on Pharmaceutical Research Expenditures: A Dynamic Approach." *Economic Enquiry*, 21, 115-128.

_____ (1984). "The Effect of U.S. Pharmaceutical Regulation on New Introductions." In *Pharmaceutical Economics*, Bjorn Lindgren (Ed.). Stockholm: Swedish Institute for Health Economics, 191-205.

Wills, J., A.C. Samli, and L. Jacobs (1991). "Developing Global Products and Marketing Strategies: A Construct and Research Agenda." *Journal of the Academy of Marketing Sciences*, 19(1), 1-10.

Yoshikawa, A. (1989). "The Other Drug War: U.S.-Japan Trade in Pharmaceuticals." *California Management Review*, (Winter), 76-90.

Young, J.H. (1982). *Public Policy and Drug Innovation*, Wisconsin: American Institute of the History of Pharmacy.

Index

Page numbers followed by the letter "f" indicate figures; those followed by the letter "t" indicate tables.